HOLISTIC HEALING
A CHRISTIAN APPROACH

HOLISTIC HEALING

A Christian Approach

Pat Collins CM

columba
BOOKS

First published in 2020 by

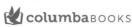 columbaBOOKS

23 Merrion Square North, Dublin 2
www.columbabooks.com

ISBN: 978-1-78218-375-4

Set in Adobe Garamond Pro 11/14 and Cinzel
Cover and book design by Alba Esteban | Columba Books

Cover Image: Christ healing a group of sick people. Engraving by A.
Schaufele, 1851. CC BY (https://creativecommons.org/licenses/by/4.0)
Source: Wikimedia Commons.

Printed by ScanBook, Sweden.

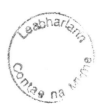

"Grant to your servants to speak your word with all boldness, while you stretch out your hand to heal"

(Acts 4:29-30)

CONTENTS

Foreword.. *9*

Preface *17*

CHAPTER 1. *Healing and the New Evangelisation*...................... *24*

CHAPTER 2. *Holistic Healing – Body, Mind & Spirit*................. *31*

CHAPTER 3. *Did Jesus Exercise the Charism of Faith*................. *38*

CHAPTER 4. *The Things I Do, You Will Do* *44*

CHAPTER 5. *Spiritual Healing* *49*

CHAPTER 6. *Deliverance & Spiritual Healing* *55*

CHAPTER 7. *Inner Healing* *61*

CHAPTER 8. *Relieving Depression* *68*

CHAPTER 9. *Ministering Inner Healing* *77*

CHAPTER 10. *The Father Wound* *85*

CHAPTER 11. *The Father Wound and False Images of God*.......... *91*

CHAPTER 12. *The Mother Wound*.................................. *98*

CHAPTER 13. *Healing the Father & Mother Wound*................. *104*

CHAPTER 14. *Prayer for Physical Healing*.......................... *110*

CHAPTER 15. *Expectant Faith and Healing*......................... *116*

CHAPTER 16. *Growing in Expectant Faith* *123*

CHAPTER 17. *Discerning God's Will in Healing* *129*

CHAPTER 18. *Healing and the Anointing of the Sick* *136*

CHAPTER 19. *Healing and the Eucharist* *143*

CHAPTER 20. *Some Protocols for Healing Prayer* *151*

CHAPTER 21. *Healing Services* *157*

CHAPTER 22. *Homily Notes on Holistic Healing* *167*

CHAPTER 23. *The Mystery of Suffering* *172*

CHAPTER 24. *Reflections on the Pandemic* *180*

CHAPTER 25. *Consecration of One's Hands for Healing Ministry* ... *190*

APPENDIX ONE.
Spiritual Warfare Prayer *194*

APPENDIX TWO.
Forgiveness prayer *198*

APPENDIX THREE.
Blessing of Olive Oil & Water in Honour of St Vincent de Paul *201*

Recommended Reading *205*

FOREWORD

During my teenage years I intended, for a time, to study medicine in the Royal College of Surgeons in Dublin with a view to becoming a doctor. The medical profession attracted me because I thought that a life devoted to healing the sick, like two of my mother's brothers, would have been really worthwhile. However, with the passage of time it became clear to me that my true vocation was to become a priest like three of my father's brothers. So I dropped the idea of becoming a doctor and decided to become a priest. I entered the seminary in 1963.

During my time studying theology, I particularly enjoyed the classes on scripture. However, when I read the Gospels and the Acts of the Apostles, I was struck by the fact that there seemed to be such a disparity between what happened in the early church, such as healings and miracles, and what was happening, or should I say, not happening in the contemporary Church. I can remember one of my priest lecturers saying that I was a dreamer with unrealistic expectations. He said he was worried about my future in priestly ministry because my boredom threshold was low. He said that in reality a good deal of priestly work would be humdrum and routine. In spite of what he said, I continued to dream.

In 1974, three years after my ordination, when I was still a relatively young man, I had the good fortune to join the Charismatic Renewal. I was baptised in the Holy Spirit and discovered the wonderful existence of the gifts of the Spirit, one of which was the gift of healing. In 1979 an international charismatic conference was held in the Royal Dublin Society. It was attended by about 20,000 people from all over the world. At one point I met the priest who had said years beforehand that I was an unrealistic dreamer. We had a cup of coffee together. In the course of our conversation he said something I have never forgotten, "Pat during your time in the seminary I really thought that your expectations were far too high, but seeing what is happening here, I realise that you have found what you were looking for and that your dream has come true." He was right. Sadly, that priest was murdered some time later by a drug addict, and apparently died with words of forgiveness on his lips.

A lot of water has passed under the bridge since then. Happily, I have never regretted my choice to become a priest and I can't remember ever being bored. In retrospect, I'm not at all sure whether I would have been a good doctor. However, I have found that, as a priest, my desire to help the sick has been satisfied by means of the healing ministry. By the grace of God, I have had the joy of seeing many people being healed over the years. Now that I'm in the autumn of my life, I have decided to write a book on the subject of Christian healing, one which draws on all that I have learned and experienced over a few decades.

I have been fortunate because I have enjoyed relatively good health down through the years. That said, I did develop a bad case of angina when I was about fifty. It was disconcerting because if I walked up a slope or had to climb a flight of stairs I would suffer from a scary feeling of chest pain. Over the years, people prayed for me, and I received the sacrament of the anointing of the sick on a few occasions. I don't quite know why, but my angina has disappeared completely, and now twenty five years later I have no problem either walking up slopes or climbing stairs. I can recall telling an Indian nun, who was a medical doctor, about what had happened and asking her why my angina had ended, and she replied, "Pat I'm surprised that you ask the question, it seems clear to me that the Lord has healed you so that you can go on evangelising in his name." As someone who has experienced divine healing myself, it is my fondest desire to help other people to experience that same healing in their lives.

It has to be recognised however, that in our secular culture there are many people, who because of their rationalistic presuppositions of a scientific nature, would deny the possibility that I could have been healed by God. In 1965 Dietrich Von Hildebrand, a well known Catholic philosopher, had a private audience with St Paul VI, during which he said, "Your Holiness, you must realise that the Church is going through the worst crisis in history, worse than the Protestant Reformation."[1] Then von Hildebrand continued: "What has taken place is that people have lost sight of the supernatural." Around the same time, Langdon Gilkey, a well known Lutheran theologian in America, wrote a book entitled, *Catholicism Confronts Modernity: A Protestant View*.[2] In it he acknowledged that the Catholic Church was experiencing a transitional crisis. He noted, with approval, that one of the main causes was, "the dissolution of the understanding of the supernatural as the central religious category." As a result he felt that Catholics were tending to reinterpret transcendent truths in worldly or naturalistic ways rather than in the traditional supernatural ones.

Those with a reductionist point of view like French novelist Emile Zola (1840-1902), will reject any supernatural explanation of healing no matter what evidence there is to the contrary. In the 1890s Zola visited Lourdes on a few occasions. He dismissed the story of the apparitions of Our Lady to St Bernadette and the claim that many people were cured in the baths. During one of his visits Zola met a girl of eighteen named Marie Lemarchand who was afflicted with three seemingly incurable diseases: an advanced stage of lupus, pulmonary tuberculosis, and leg ulcerations the size of an adult's hand. Zola described the girl's face on the way to Lourdes as being eaten away by the lupus, "Her face was a frightful distorted mass of matter and oozing blood." The girl went into the baths and emerged completely cured. One of the doctors who was present later wrote, "On her return from the baths I at once

---

1   Dr Alice Von Hildebrand, "The Secular War on the Supernatural" https://www.romancatholicman.com/secular-war-supernatural-alice-von-hildebrand/
2   (New York: Seabury Press, 1975).

followed her to the hospital. I recognized her although her face was entirely changed."[3]

The doctors who examined her could also find nothing wrong with her lungs, both of which had been infected with tuberculosis, causing the patient to cough and spit blood. Although Zola witnessed the miracle he refused to accept it as anything other than a psychosomatic event. He stated, "I don't believe in miracles. Even if all the sick in Lourdes were cured in one moment I would not believe in them."[4] As G. K. Chesterton said rightly in his book, *Orthodoxy*, "The believers in miracles accept them because they have evidence for them. The disbelievers in miracles deny them because *they have a doctrine against them*."[5] Like Zola, many people in our secular, post-truth society, have decided on the basis of their secular prejudices that supernatural healing cannot and does not occur.

Whether one has, or has not a sense of the supernatural, has a big bearing on the subject matter of this book. When people suffer from mental health problems and sicknesses, those who espouse a naturalistic point of view will try to understand and cure them in purely human terms. They maintain that the only form of healing that is possible is the kind that is brought about solely by means of medical and psychiatric treatments. Besides resorting to those human means, Christians believe that there is abundant evidence that God can and does heal people in supernatural ways. Bible scholar, Craig S Keener has provided persuasive evidence of this in his scholarly two volume, *Miracles: The Credibility of New Testament Accounts*, which not only takes a critical look at the miracles in biblical times but also at numerous examples in the modern world.[6]

---

3 Quoted by Karl Keating in *The Usual Suspects: Answering Anti-Catholic Fundamentalists* (San Francisco: Ignatius Press, 2000), 138.

4 Quoted by Matthew Archbold in "I Am a Miracle Man" *National Catholic Register. https://www.ncregister.com/blog/matthew-archbold/i_am_a_miracle_man*

5 *Orthodoxy* (New York: John Lane, 1909)

6 (Grand Rapids: Baker, 2011).

This book is addressed to those who are open in mind and heart to the possibility of divine healing. I should acknowledge that Christianity not only talks about the healing of people, increasingly and quite rightly it speaks about the healing of the natural world which has been ravaged by irresponsible human activity, which among other things is causing global warming. Although Pope Francis drew attention to this important subject in his encyclical *Laudato Si* (On the Care of Our Common Home) I will not be dealing with it in this book.

I want to thank the many men and women with whom I have run healing services, over a period of forty six years in many different countries. Not only have they edified me by their compassion and faith, they have also taught me a great deal about the ministry. I want to offer a particular word of gratitude to Sr. Jane Ford of the Holy Faith Sisters who has helped me in the preparation of this book. I also want to express my appreciation for the help of the members of the New Springtime Community, who assisted in many practical ways to run a twenty week course on the subject of healing in Donnybrook, Dublin. I also want to say a big "thank you" to the wonderful men and women who attended the course, asked perceptive questions, and offered helpful feedback. May the Lord bless each and every one of them as they seek to bring Christ's healing to others. This book is dedicated to Jana Ungerová and Vašek Čáp in gratitude for being my interpreters and collaborators during my many visits to the Czech Republic in recent years.

A PRAYER TO BE SAID BEFORE READING THIS BOOK

Come, Holy Spirit, Divine Creator, source of light and fountain of wisdom. As I read this book on healing grant me the ability to pay sustained attention to its contents, a penetrating and reflective mind to understand them, a retentive memory to recall what is important, and the lucidity to comprehend the nature of the gift of healing, the motives I have for experiencing and exercising it, and the practical means at my disposal for doing so in my daily life. Guide the beginning of my reading, direct its progress, and bring it to a successful completion in order that I may bring solace and peace to those who suffer and thereby bring glory to your holy name. This I ask through Jesus Christ, true God and true man, living and reigning with you and the Father, forever and ever. Amen.

PREFACE

Like many older Catholics I grew up as the Counter-Reformation was coming to an end. It had held sway from the end of the Council of Trent in 1563 to the end of the second Vatican Council. I can remember my mother telling me in 1959 that Pope John XXIII was going to convene a gathering of all the bishops of the Church. When I asked her what the Council aimed to do, she said, "I think it is going to try to heal the rift between the Catholic and Protestant Churches." She wasn't far wrong. The 1964 *Decree on Ecumenism* began with these words, "The restoration of unity among all Christians is one of the principal concerns of the Second Vatican Council... division openly contradicts the will of Christ, scandalizes the world, and damages the holy cause of preaching the Gospel to every creature." I think that the connection between inter-church unity and effective evangelisation is a vital one. The extent to which unity is lacking in and between churches is the extent to which their evangelisation will lack credibility and effectiveness.

When I was ordained in 1971, a few years after the ending of the Council, I was sent to St Patrick's College in Armagh to teach. The troubles were at their height in Northern Ireland. During the next three years I felt a growing spiritual unease within that context of animosity and violence. I knew something was missing in my spiritual life, but couldn't put my finger on what it was. On Feb 4th 1974 I heard Rev Cecil Kerr, a Church of Ireland clergyman, speaking about the fact that Jesus is our peace who breaks down the dividing wall of division between Jews and Gentiles, Catholics and Protestants. Quite frankly, his inspired words moved me to tears. I wanted to know the Lord in the way he already did. I told him that I was looking for a new awareness of God in my life. He responded by reading a memorable passage from Eph 3:14-20 which expressed exactly what I was seeking. Then he began to pray over me, firstly in English, then in tongues. Suddenly, and effortlessly, I too began to pray fluently in tongues. I knew with great conviction that Jesus loved me and accepted me as I was. As a result of that religious awakening, I was fully persuaded that the Lord was not only strongly at work within me to will and to do his good pleasure he was also at work, in the same way, in members of other churches.

Afterwards Cecil Kerr and I became great friends. He used to say that there would be no genuine reconciliation without renewal in the Holy Spirit, and no genuine renewal in the Holy Spirit without reconciliation. Over the years I repeatedly witnessed the fact that once Catholics and Protestants were baptised in the Holy Spirit they had a God prompted desire both to work for inter-church reconciliation and to carry out the great commission by evangelising separately and together. During those years I made an important discovery about the nature of evangelisation, one that has influenced me ever since.

Those who evangelise seek to share the message of salvation through faith in Jesus. According to Leon-Dufour's *Dictionary of the New Testament*, the Greek word for save is *sozo*. It is derived from *saos* meaning healthy.[1] In other words, salvation and healing are two sides of the same coin of grace. The two meanings are virtually interchangeable and synonymous in the gospels. For example, when Jesus healed people physically, he often said "your faith has saved you" (cf. Mk 10:52; Lk 17:19; 18:42). The same inter-connection is evident in Jm 5:13-16 which is about the sacrament of the anointing of the sick. It asserts that, "the prayer of faith will save the one who is sick." In this text the word save can be simultaneously understood in terms of spiritual salvation and the possibility of physical healing. So healing is integral to evangelisation and should be normative for all evangelisers.

Church history makes it clear that in the early centuries the notions of salvation and healing were closely interrelated in theory

1   (San Francisco: Harper & Row, 1980), 361.

and practice. For example, Origen (185-284) wrote, "the name of Jesus can still remove distractions from the minds of men, and expel demons, and also take away diseases."[2] In his book, *Christianising the Roman Empire*, Ramsay MacMullen argued that it was miracles, including healings that more than anything else drew converts to the early Church.[3] But somewhere along the line the connection between salvation and healing became separated. Morton Kelsey described in detail how this happened in his book, *Healing and Christianity*,[4] as did Francis Mac Nutt in his *The Nearly Perfect Crime: How the Church Almost Killed the Ministry of Healing*.[5]

Over time in the early Church the institutional elements tended to replace the more charismatic ones. A mistaken cessationist theory argued that the charisms, including healing and miracle working, were given to get the early Church up and running, but were withdrawn by God when its structures and sacraments were in operation. So although we expected the sacraments to be means of saving grace, up to the mid twentieth century, we did not really expect them to bring about any kind of physical or emotional healing. Even the anointing of the sick was seen as a sacrament preparing people spiritually for death. Because the charisms mentioned in 1 Cor 12:8-10 no longer seemed to be in evidence, neither priests or lay people laid hands on the sick in the expectation that they would be healed. That said some vestiges of non-sacramental healing survived down the years.

Firstly, there were saints who were notable for their healing powers such as Francis of Paola, Vincent Ferrer, and Francis of Assisi. If you read *The Life Of Saint Francis of Assisi*,[6] a biography which was written by his fellow Franciscan, St Bonaventure, you will find in chapter twelve, entitled, "Of the efficacy of his preaching, and

---

2   *Contra Celsus*, Book 1, Chapter 67.
3   (New Haven: Yale University Press, 1984)
4   (London: SCM, 1973)
5   (Grand Rapids: Chosen, 2005)
6   (New York: Harper Collins, 2009)

of his gift of healing," that there are numerous examples of the fact that he not only proclaimed the coming of God's kingdom, Francis demonstrated its coming by means of his numerous healings. It struck me that Bonaventure seemed to be saying that Jesus Christ had walked the earth once more in and through the life and ministry of his servant Francis.

Secondly, there were occasional reports of ordinary lay people healing the sick. I discovered a fascinating example in *The Journey & Ordeal of Cabeza De Vaca: His Account of the Disastrous First European Exploration of the American Southwest.* Between 1528 and 1536 De Vaca and three other Spaniards survived shipwreck in America. As they wandered for eight years through the southern part of the continent they told Indians they met about their belief in the Christian God. When the natives asked them for healing prayers the Spanish adventurers responded. De Vaca said, "Our method was to bless the sick, breathe upon them, recite a *Pater noster* and *Ave Maria* and pray earnestly to God our Lord for their recovery." Later he reported, "We all prayed the best we could for their health; we knew that only through him would these people help us so we might emerge from this unhappy existence. And he bestowed health so bountifully that every patient got up the following morning as sound and strong as if he had never had an illness."[7]

Francis MacNutt says that, surprisingly, for seven hundred years or so, in England and France, it was believed that the "royal touch" of the King, who was the Lord's anointed, could result in healing.[8] Apparently the monarchs in both countries used to conduct healing services a few times a year, during which not only were large numbers of people prayed with, apparently many of them were healed. The people believed that the king could heal in virtue of his anointed role rather than his personal holiness of life.

Thirdly, other forms of healing tended to be relegated to the margins of the Church, such as visiting shrines like Lourdes, blessing

7   (New York: Dover, 2003), 64; 87.
8   *The Nearly Perfect Crime,* op. cit., 133-137.

with relics of the saints, having recourse to folk healers who were believed to have cures for specific ailments such as broken bones, shingles, and warts.[9] In Ireland, and some other countries, there was the curious belief that the seventh son of a seventh son would be endowed with healing powers.[10]

An important change was agreed at the Second Vatican Council between 1962-1965. Following a debate of historical significance, the bishops chose to include a paragraph in the *Constitution of the Church* which spoke about the potential role the charisms of the Holy Spirit, including those of healing and miracle working. They described the edifying effect they could have if God chose to restore them to the faithful. Par. 12 stated, "The manifestation of the Spirit is given to everyone for profit. These charisms, whether they be the more outstanding or the more simple and widely diffused, are to be received with thanksgiving and consolation for they are perfectly suited to and useful for the needs of the Church." These words anticipated, in a prophetic way, the advent of the Catholic Charismatic Renewal Movement in 1967, firstly in the USA, and then in one country after another around the world. As a result, all the gifts mentioned in 1 Cor 12:8-10 were restored, after a lapse of sixteen hundred years or more, and widely distributed among clerical and lay members alike.

Speaking about this phenomenon Joseph Ratzinger - later Pope Benedict XVI - said, "In the heart of a world adversely affected by rationalistic skepticism, a new experience of the Holy Spirit has come about, amounting to a worldwide renewal movement. What the New Testament describes with reference to the charisms as visible signs of the coming of the Spirit is no longer merely ancient, past history: this history is becoming a burning reality today."[11]

9   Cf. Nora Smyth, RSCJ *Going for the Cure: Traditional Healing in Armagh Area* (Armagh, Smyth, 2003).

10   *The Nearly Perfect Crime,* op. cit., 136.

11   Ratzinger and Messori, *The Ratzinger Report* (San Francisco: Ignatius Press, 1985), 151.

Some years later, Pope Benedict XVI, said in his book, *Jesus of Nazareth*, that "Healing is an essential dimension of the apostolic mission and of the Christian faith in general. It can even be said that Christianity is a 'therapeutic religion, a religion of healing.'"[12] In an interesting interview Pope Francis said in like manner, "The thing the church needs most today is the ability to heal wounds and to warm the hearts of the faithful; it needs nearness, proximity. I see the church as a field hospital after battle."[13]

By the year 2000 it was estimated that about a hundred million Catholics had shared in the charismatic experience. In that same year the Congregation for the Doctrine of the Faith published a significant document, entitled *Instruction on Prayers of Healing*. Section five bore the heading, "The charism of healing in the present-day context." While it established disciplinary norms to regulate the conduct of the healing ministry, what is notable is the fact that it affirmed that the charism of healing can indeed lead to genuine cures of different kinds. During my long involvement with the Charismatic Renewal, not only have I witnessed many people being healed, I have been blessed to have seen a number of men and women being healed when I prayed with them. That said the *Instruction* added the following cautionary observation, "not even the most intense prayer obtains the healing of all sicknesses. So it is that St. Paul had to learn from the Lord that, "my grace is enough for you; my power is made perfect in weakness" (2 Cor 12:9)." We will return to this topic in chapter twenty two.

I belong to the New Springtime Community in Dublin which is devoted to evangelising and training evangelisers. We conducted a twelve week course on deliverance ministry in 2018- 2019.[14] It was popular and we intended to run it a second time. However, during one of our prayer times, when about ten of us were on pilgrimage

---

12 (San Francisco: Ignatius Press, 2007), 176.
13 Interview with *America*, September 2013.
14 Pat Collins, C.M., *Freedom From Evil Spirits: Released From Fear, Addiction and the Devil* (Dublin: Veritas, 2019).

in Međugorje, the Lord seemed to say that instead of running the deliverance course again, we should run a course on Christian healing, one aspect of which could be deliverance. In obedience to that word of guidance we ran a twenty week course on healing from late September 2019 until Spring 2020. Ironically it was interrupted by the coronavirus (Covid-19) pandemic. This book had its roots in that venture and the constructive feedback it evoked. It is my hope that it will prove, to be a practical guide which will aid its readers to understand and experience healing in their own lives as well as equipping them, and others, to know how to minister spiritual, emotional and physical healing to the suffering and wounded people of our time.

CHAPTER ONE

....

HEALING AND THE NEW EVANGELISATION

The New Evangelisation is the re-evangelisation of those who in spite of being baptised and confirmed are not fully converted to the Lord. In the working document for the 2012 Synod on the New Evangelisation, the concept was defined in par. 85 as follows, "The phrase 'new evangelisation' designates pastoral outreach to those who no longer practice the Christian faith." When the Synod was over Cardinal Donald Wuerl, its Secretary General, defined the subject succinctly: "At its heart the New Evangelisation is the re-proposing of the encounter with the risen Lord, his Gospel and his Church to those who no longer find the Church's message engaging." Here we see that the essence of the New Evangelisation is about relationship with the Risen Jesus and helping people to move from knowing about the person of Jesus to knowing him in person.[1]

Following his baptism at the Jordan, Acts 1:1 tells us that Jesus did two main things, he began 'to *do* and to *teach*'. In other words, he *proclaimed* the Good News of God's unconditional mercy and love, especially to the poor and *demonstrated* the reality of that Good News, especially by means of healings, exorcisms and miracles. Proclamation and demonstration were inseparable. When Jesus proclaimed the Good News of God's unconditional and unrestricted mercy and love, he announced the fact that the curse of sin was being lifted as an unmerited gift. The Jews believed that illness

---

1   On the new evangelisation see Pat Collins, C.M. *Encountering Jesus: New Evangelisation in Practice* (Luton: New Life, 2017).

and handicaps were the penalty of sin. So as a sign that the curse of sin had indeed been lifted, Jesus removed its penalty by healing the sick and driving out evil spirits. All the evangelists regarded the healings and exorcisms not only as an integral part of the message itself, they were presented simply as the good news in action.

During his public ministry Jesus instructed the apostles to do the same. He said to them and all believers, "Truly, truly, I say to you, whoever believes in me will also do the works that I do; and greater works than these will he do, because I am going to the Father. Whatever you ask in my name, this I will do, that the Father may be glorified in the Son" (Jn 14:12-13). Implicit in that promise was the assertion that the disciples would not only be able to preach like Jesus but would also heal the sick on his behalf.[2] Like him, they were to *proclaim* and *demonstrate* the coming of the Kingdom of God. In Mk 16:15-19 we read: "He said to them, 'Go into all the world and preach the good news to all creation. Whoever believes and is baptised will be saved, but whoever does not believe will be condemned. And these signs will accompany those who believe: In my name they will drive out demons... they will place their hands on sick people, and they will get well.'"

When one reads the Acts and especially the earlier epistles of Paul, it becomes apparent that having been baptised in the Spirit the apostles did carry out the Lord's instructions. They not only proclaimed the Good News, they demonstrated it in deeds of power including healing. Acts 2:43 testifies that having preached the gospel message, "Many wonders and signs were done through the apostles." In Acts 8:6-7 we are told about the evangelisation of the deacon Philip, "With one accord, the crowds paid attention to what was said by Philip when they heard it and saw the signs he was doing. For unclean spirits, crying out in a loud voice, came out of many possessed people, and many paralyzed and crippled people were cured."

2   Cf. Pat Collins, CM., "Claiming the Promises of Scripture" in *Word and Spirit: Intimations of a New Springtime* (Dublin: Columba, 2011), 104-125.

There is clear evidence also that the charisms were exercised in the first centuries of Christianity. The early church fathers and theologians such as, Irenaeus, Justin Martyr, Origen and Tertullian all spoke about charismatic manifestations. However, for a number of reasons, healing began to die out in the first three centuries, but not totally. St. Augustine (354-430) gives us an insight into the late 4th and early 5th century. In the earlier part of his life, he believed that all miracles ended with the Apostles but his view was changed as a result of many miracles that occurred during a powerful revival throughout the churches of North Africa, so that he wrote in *The City of God*, "For even now miracles are wrought in the name of Christ, whether by his sacraments or by the prayers and relics of his saints."[3] What is noticeable in this quotation, however, is the fact that there is no reference to the charisms of healing or miracle working.

As has already been noted in the introduction, by the 3rd century the emphasis shifted from the charisms to the role of the institutional church, its sacraments and rituals. Priests and people expected the Spirit to be manifested by the witness of lives well lived, in deeds of mercy and in action for justice, but not by unusual charismatic activity. In the 13th century, St Thomas Aquinas taught that canonised saints were the only exception to this rule, both during their lifetimes and after their deaths. He wrote: "True miracles cannot be wrought save by the power of God, because God works them … in proof of a person's holiness which God desires to propose as an example of virtue." For example, in the 14th century, Thomas's fellow Dominican, St. Vincent Ferrer, exercised many of the spiritual gifts. If he preached in his native dialect, he was understood by those of other nationalities. He is reputed to have performed countless healings and miracles including the raising of 32 people from the dead.[4]

---

3   *City of God* book xxii, chapt., 8.
4   Cf. "The canonization process for St Vincent Ferrer" in *Medieval Hagiography: An Anthology* (London: Routledge, 2000), 781-803.

Baptism in the Spirit and healing

Pope John XXIII prayed before the Second Vatican Council for the renewal of the Church: 'O Holy Spirit, renew your wonders in this our day, as by a new Pentecost.' In 1967 his prayer was answered when Catholics began to be baptised in the Spirit. This kind of spiritual awakening can be described as follows, "It is a life-transforming experience of the love of God the Father poured into one's heart by the Holy Spirit, received through a surrender to the Lordship of Jesus Christ. It brings alive sacramental baptism and confirmation, deepens communion with God and with fellow Christians, enkindles evangelistic fervour and equips a person with charisms for service and mission."[5] It is worth mentioning in this context that speaking to a gathering of members of the Charismatic Movement in 2019, Pope Francis said, "What does the Pope expect of you? I expect this movement to share baptism in the Spirit with *everyone* in the Church."[6] Over the years experience has taught us that it is only those who have received this in-filling of the Spirit who exercise the more exceptional charisms, such as healing and miracle working.

Classification and use of the Charisms

Paul's theology of the gifts was an expression of his pastoral experience, and not of his theological speculation. So when he listed the charisms in 1 Cor 12:8-10, he probably did so in the light of his involvement in evangelisation, e.g., in Corinth. Following St. Thomas Aquinas I would suggest, however, that they can be classified in the following way.

1) There are charisms of *revelation* that enable the believer to know the presence, word and will of the Lord, e.g., wisdom, knowledge, prophetic revelation, words of knowledge, interpretation of messages in tongues.

---

5   *Baptism in the Spirit* (Luton: New Life 2012), 15.
6   Pope Francis in *CHARIS Magazine*, special issue No. 1, 2019, 5-6. www. charis.international

2) There are charisms of *proclamation* that enable the believer to preach, teach or share the Good News, e.g., utterance of words of wisdom and knowledge, prophecy proclaimed, utterances in tongues.

3) There are charisms of *demonstration* which manifest the Good News, e.g., by means of liberating deeds of power such as, healings, miracle working and deliverance from evil spirits which are made possible by the charism of faith.

It is worth mentioning at this point that, in its official teaching on the charisms, the Church makes a number of encouraging and empowering points which lay people, in particular, need to know. Firstly, grace comes to us not only through sacraments and clerical ministry, but also through the charisms of the Spirit, including the list mentioned in 1 Cor 12:8-10, e.g., healing.[7] Secondly, lay people have a right to exercise their charisms. This right comes from their baptism into Christ and not from the clergy.[8] Thirdly, lay people have a duty to use their charisms for the good and up-building of the Church and the world.[9] Fourthly, bishops and clergy should test the charisms to see that they are genuine and used for the common good. However, they should be careful not to quench the Spirit by an arbitrary use of authority.[10]

Relevance of the charisms today

Sadly, we are living at a time when millions of Europeans have drifted away from the Church. Many of them have little or no sense of a supernatural realm beyond their everyday sense experience. When Christians can demonstrate the truth of the Good News message by means of supernatural deeds of power, such as healings and miracles, which manifest the presence and power of

7 *Lumen Gentium # 12.*
8 *Apostolicam Actuositatem # 3*
9 *Apostolicam Actuositatem # 3*
10 *Lumen Gentium # 12; Apostolicam Actuositatem # 3.*

the Lord, many open minded people will come to have faith in Jesus Christ.

In the course of launching Cardinal Suenen's book, *A New Pentecost?* in 1974, Pope Paul VI said in some impromptu remarks, "How wonderful it would be if the Lord would again pour out the charisms in increased abundance, in order to make the Church fruitful, beautiful and marvellous, and to enable it to win the attention and astonishment of the profane and secularised world."[11] Sometime later Pope Francis talked in a similar vein about the role of the charisms in par. 130 of *The Joy of the Gospel*, "They are not an inheritance, safely secured and entrusted to a small group for safekeeping [e. g. the members of the Charismatic Renewal], rather they are gifts of the Spirit integrated into the body of the Church, drawn to the centre which is Christ and then channelled into an evangelising impulse."

In an article entitled, "The Charisms and the New Evangelisation" by Cardinal Danneels, the Belgian primate echoed those papal sentiments when he wrote, "In times of crisis like today, the Spirit multiplies its gifts." A little later he added, "The more the life of the people of God is harsh, the more God grants his gifts. What would be the particular gifts today which the Lord gives us? Would it not be faith which moves mountains, which brings about healings and which thus gives weight to the proclamation of the gospel?"[12]

Thankfully the healing spoken about by St Paul VI and Cardinal Danneels is alive and well in the contemporary world. Here are three short examples that come to mind as I write. Two or three years ago, a priest from the Czech Republic visited me. In the course of conversation he thanked me. He explained that he had been suffering from Crone's Disease, and that I had anointed him at a healing service in Zeliv. He reported that soon afterwards, a doctor had confirmed the fact that the disease was no longer active

---

11 *Pope Paul and the Spirit,* ed. by Edward O' Connor (Notre Dame: Ave Maria Press, 1978), 210-212.

12 *Goodnews* magazine (Jan/Feb 2007)

in his life. More recently I was due to conduct a healing service in a church in Belfast. Beforehand a Protestant man came to see me and a companion of mine. He told us that he was suffering from cancer and asked for prayer. We ministered to him and discovered some time later that his cancer had disappeared. When we went to the Belfast healing service, I got a word of knowledge for a man who spoke to me. I urged him to see a doctor to get his blood checked. He did what I had said, and was saved from dying as a result of his blood disease being diagnosed and treated.

Conclusion

The flowering of the charisms in the late twentieth and early twenty first centuries has been a providential blessing of great significance. Just as Jesus received the charisms at his baptism and the disciples received them at Pentecost, so modern Christians receive the gifts of the Spirit in order, like Jesus and the disciples, to engage in effective evangelisation. We can end this chapter with some words spoken by Pope John Paul II, Pentecost 1998, at an historical gathering of new ecclesial movements and communities in Rome, "Today, I would like to cry out to all of you gathered here in St. Peter's Square and to all Christians, open yourselves docilely to the gifts of the Spirit! Accept gracefully and obediently the charisms which the Spirit never ceases to bestow on us! Do not forget that every charism is given for the common good, that is, for the benefit of the whole Church."[13] Among those wonderful charisms, of course, is the gift of healings (cf. Mk 16:18; 1 Cor 12:9).

13 http://www.vatican.va/content/john-paul-ii/en/speeches/1998/may/docu-
ments/hf_jp-ii_spe_19980530_riflessioni.html

Chapter Two

....

Holistic Healing – Body, Mind & Spirit

A foundation stone is a large block that is put in position at the start of work on a public building. We begin this chapter with an interesting and important quotation about the Biblical anthropology implicit in 1 Thess 5:23. It will be the cornerstone, not only of this chapter, but also of the holistic approach to healing informing this book. St Paul wrote, "Now may the God of peace himself sanctify you completely, and may your whole *spirit* and *soul* and *body* be kept blameless at the coming of our Lord Jesus Christ. " Notice that Paul thinks that a human being is a trinity, so to speak, consisting of

1) Spirit, (*psyche* in Greek), i.e., mind, which consists of conscious and unconscious experience, emotions, memory, will etc.

2) Soul, (*pneuma* in Greek), i.e., that part of a human which can only be satisfied by relationship with the God of ultimate meaning and love.

3) Body, (*soma* in Greek), i.e., the fleshly part of us which relates us to the material world and the people around us.[1]

It is important to note that St Paul was not stating that a human being is made up of three parts but rather that there are three interrelated aspects to the human person. That being so, they interact with one another. For example, nowadays doctors talk about psychosomatic

---

1   For an excellent discussion of this topic see, George Montague, "Body, Soul and Spirit," in *Riding the Wind: Learning the Ways of the Spirit* (Ann Arbor: Word of Life, 1977), 26-39.

illnesses, i.e., disorders of the body which are directly, or indirectly influenced by a person's mental and emotional state. For instance, it is thought that up to 85% of physical illness is probably directly or indirectly caused by unhealthy levels of chronic stress. Acute, unrelieved stress can lead directly to dangerously high blood pressure which in turn can cause heart attacks and strokes, and indirectly to a weakened immune system which renders a person vulnerable to all kinds of infections and diseases, such as cancer. The placebo effect is another example of the power of the mind to influence the body. It is a beneficial effect produced by a placebo, i.e., an inactive drug or treatment, which cannot be attributed to the properties of the placebo itself, and must therefore be due to the patient's belief in that treatment.

Christians believe that besides the body and mind there is the soul, that part of us which is hard wired for religious experience. Writing about it Blaise Paschal stated, "There is a God-shaped vacuum in the heart of each person which cannot be satisfied by any created thing but only by God the Creator, made known through Jesus Christ."[2] In other words, the soul is that part of us which can only be satisfied by conscious awareness of the "higher power," to use the terminology of Alcoholics Anonymous, or the "numinous" to use a phrase made popular by Rudolf Otto, author of *The Idea of the Holy*.[3]

Just as the mind can have an effect on the body, so the soul can have a positive or negative effect, as we shall see in a later chapter, on both the mind and the body. George Montague has written in *Riding the Wind*, "If the psyche has such an influence on the body, might not the spirit in turn have a powerful influence on the psyche and through the psyche on the body as well? If we can speak of psychosomatic diseases, might we not also speak of pneuma-psychosomatic diseases? Such diseases have psychic and somatic effects but their roots are really in the underdeveloped or constricted

2   Paraphrase of *Pensées* VII (425).
3   (London: Oxford University Press, 1923).

pneuma."[4] Montague went on to add, that his own experience, both personal and pastoral, had convinced him that spiritually caused diseases are common and that many psychic and somatic healings can be accomplished simply through healing of the *pneuma* or soul. We will revisit this point in more depth in subsequent chapters.

It follows from this threefold understanding of the human person that there are three main interrelated forms of healing:

1) *Spiritual healing,* i.e., releasing what has been referred to as the underdeveloped, constricted, or frustrated self or soul.

2) *Inner healing,* i.e., healing of hurting memories, troubled emotions and psychological problems, thereby enabling troubled people to experience peace.

3) *Physical healing,* i.e., healing such things as injuries, diseases, infections and handicaps.

From a Christian point of view, integral healing is like a three legged stool. If any one leg is too short or missing it will not be able to stand. Sadly, in Western secular culture, many people either deny or ignore the fact that we have a soul. As a result they understand healing solely in psychosomatic terms. Currently, it is quite noticeable that the need for good mental health is a constant topic of discussion in the mass media because so many people struggle with all kinds of issues such as anxiety states, panic attacks, depression, addiction and even suicidal ideation. What is noticeable, however, is the fact that quite often such problems are understood solely in psychological and electro-chemical terms, while the role of the soul, and its need for ultimate meaning is often overlooked or denied. Christians on the other hand will sometimes see a link between the spiritual state of the person's soul and his or her mental health. For instance, a Christian healer might have reason to think that a person's mental agitation is being adversely effected by oppression by evil spirits. If that oppression is lifted, the healing powers of the

---

4   *Riding the Wind,* op. cit., 36.

mind can not only be released but they can be assisted by means of medication and psychotherapy. It strikes me that Jesus adopted this three legged holistic approach to salvation and healing.

Jesus' Holistic Approach to Healing

A. Spiritual Healing

Jesus healed people spiritually by offering to lift the curse of sin from those who trusted in him and his words of love. Those who changed their way of thinking and believed in him experienced the forgiveness of all their wrongdoing in a way which was neither earned, merited, nor deserved. Surely, that kind of spiritual healing was experienced by the Samaritan woman at Jacob's well. As Jesus said to her in Jn 4:13-14, "Everyone who drinks of this water will be thirsty again, but whoever drinks of the water that I will give him will never be thirsty again. The water that I will give him will become in him a spring of water welling up to eternal life." That was a tremendous promise of transformation. Her basic problem was a spiritual one. She had never found a love that would last forever; all that she had experienced was a series of romantic loves of a fleeting kind. She was a wounded person, looking for the right thing in the wrong place. Through her meeting with Jesus,[5] the source of love, the relationship secretly released the water of everlasting spiritual life within her. Jesus empathised with her pain, affirmed her when she spoke the truth about her relationships, and revealed to her that he was the promised Messiah. The same emphasis on spiritual healing was obvious in the case of the paralysed man in Lk 5:17-39, who was let through the roof. Jesus began by healing him spiritually by forgiving him (i.e. by lifting the curse of sin) and only then did he heal him physically (i.e. by removing the penalty). I think

---

5   John mentions that the woman had five husbands, currently she was living with a man, so Jesus was the seventh significant man in her life. In the Bible, seven is the number for perfection. In meeting Jesus she had met the man of her dreams, the perfect man who could offer her everlasting love in the Holy Spirit.

that St Paul had something like this kind of healing relationship in mind when he said in Eph 3:16, "I ask God from the wealth of his glory to give you power through his Spirit to be strong in your inner selves."

Clearly, exorcism was also an important aspect of Christ's spiritual healing. He freed people from the oppression of the prince and ruler of this world, namely, the devil and his demonic spirits. 'Demonic' is the opposite to 'symbolic.' The former literally means to 'throw apart, alienate, to separate' whereas the latter means 'to throw together, to bring into unity and wholeness.' By means of his exorcisms Jesus brought an end to inner alienation and fostered unity and peace. As he said in Lk 11:20, "If I drive out demons by the finger of God, then the kingdom of God has come upon you."

B. Emotional Healing

In the New Testament Church, there was very little if any emphasis on psychology. That said it would seem that inner healing, as we understand it, was often associated with deliverance ministry, for example when Jesus restored the Gerasene demoniac to spiritual and psychological sanity and stability (cf. Mk 5:1-20). That said, there are undoubtedly examples of Jesus helping people to experience inner peace. For example in Mt 11:28-30 he said, "Come to me, all who labour and are heavy laden, and I will give you rest. Take my yoke upon you, and learn from me, for I am gentle and lowly in heart, and you will find rest for your souls. For my yoke is easy, and my burden is light." Although the parable of the Prodigal Son (Lk 15:11-32) is about mercy, St John Paul II pointed out that it is also about the way in which the Father's unconditional compassion restored his son's dignity. That was symbolised in a special way when the son was given the cloak, which was a sign of honour, and the signet ring which was a sign of sharing in his father's authority.[6] In modern terms we could say that the experience of

---

6   *Dives in Misercordia* (Rich in Mercy), Part IV, sec. 5-6.

divine mercy in those ways increased the son's self-acceptance and self-esteem. It is also significant, particularly in his post resurrection appearances, that an oft repeated greeting of Jesus was, "Peace be with you." That benediction included the notion of happiness and health of all kinds.

C. Physical Healing

The gospels recall at least 20 physical healings which Jesus performed. For example, in Mt 12:15 we read, "He withdrew from there. And great multitudes followed Him, and *He healed them all.*" It is striking that when people doubted whether Jesus was genuinely the Messiah, instead of arguing the point, he referred them to his physical healings. So when John the Baptist sent messengers to ask Jesus, "Are you the one to come after me or shall we wait for another," (Mt 11:3) Jesus responded, "Go back and report to John what you hear and see: the blind receive sight, the lame walk, those who have leprosy are cured, the deaf hear" (Mt 11:5). On another occasion Jesus said, "Believe the works, [i.e. the physical healings and miracles] that you may know and understand that the Father is in me, and I in the Father" (Jn 10:38; 14:11). In the course of his sermon on Pentecost day, St Peter referred to the healings of Jesus when he said, "Listen to these words, fellow-Israelites! Jesus of Nazareth was a man whose divine authority was clearly proven to you by all the miracles and wonders which God performed through him." (Acts 2:22). Jesus instructed the apostles to do the same. Like him, they were to proclaim and demonstrate the coming of the Kingdom of God in the way he had done.

Conclusion

The Christian life is essentially about relationship, relationship with ourselves, the world of people and nature and through both with God. At the heart of all relationship is the need for trust, i.e., faith. It is surely of great significance that Jesus said to so many people "your faith has healed you" or "made you well" (cf. Mt 9:22; Mk 5:34;

Lk 17:19; 18:42). In other words, because you trusted in me, God was able to come into your life in a healing way by the power of the Holy Spirit, the Lord and *giver of life.* In the next chapter we will ask the controversial question, did Jesus himself exercise faith, as trust in God the Father, when he healed people in body, mind or soul?

Chapter Three

....

Did Jesus Exercise the Charism of Faith?

The Gospels make it abundantly clear that faith is the key to healing. Normally it is needed both by the one who prays for healing and the one who requests healing prayer, together with any of his or her companions who are present. We Christians believe that in Christ Jesus, God has become like us in all things but sin (cf. Heb 2.17; 4.15). If that is so, can we say that, like us, Jesus needed to trust in God the Father in order to perform healings and miracles?

In our culture we say that people have faith if they believe in the existence of God. Clearly, it would be absurd to think that Jesus had that kind of faith. After all, he himself was divine. Christian faith can also be understood as the assent of mind and heart to revealed truth taught by scripture. Jesus did not have this kind of faith either. As he himself testified, "I am the... truth" (Jn 14:6). Christians also talk about saving faith, e.g., in Rom 1:17, "The righteous will live by faith." Obviously, as one who was utterly sinless and divine, Jesus didn't need to have justifying faith.

So it would seem that the Son of God did not have those common forms of faith. St Thomas Aquinas confirmed this fact when he said in one of his writings, "Faith is the evidence of things not seen." But there was nothing that was not known to Christ, according to what Peter said to him 'You know all things.' Therefore there was no faith in Christ."[1] That said, Cardinal Avery Dulles wrote in his book *The Assurance of Things Hoped For: A Theology of Christian*

---

1   *Summa Theologiae*, third part, question 7, art. 3.

Faith, that it could be said that Jesus possessed an 'archetypal faith,' i.e., an exemplary form of trust. "Even though Jesus, as the incarnate Son, did not have faith in the same sense that other beings do, he exemplifies in an eminent manner the obedience and trust that are constitutive of faith."[2] In the passion account people at the foot of the cross said of Jesus, "He trusts in God. Let God rescue him now if he wants him" (Mt 27:43). As Jesus says in Heb 2:13 "I will put my trust in him." That trust found pre-eminent expression at the very end of his life when Jesus said, "Father into your hands I commit my spirit" (Lk 23:46).

High and Low Christology

Underpinning the assertion that Jesus trusted in God is an understanding of the doctrine of the two natures in Christ, the divine and the human. Some theologians, e.g., Thomas Aquinas, emphasise the divinity of Christ, such as the fact that he was all knowing and all powerful, while many modern theologians emphasise the humanity of Christ, the fact that he emptied himself of his divine prerogatives when he became man (cf. Phil 2:7). As the Son of God, Jesus was equal in *nature* to the Father. As he said, "I and the Father are one" (Jn 10:30). But as a human being, with a human nature like ours, Jesus was subordinate in *role*. As he said, "The Father is greater than I" (Jn 14:28). That being so, Jesus was like us in *all* things but sin, and as a result "*increased* in wisdom and in stature and in favour with God and man" (Lk 2:52). As someone who was obedient to the Father (cf. Heb 10:7), he himself testified, "I did not speak on my own, but the Father who sent me commanded me to say all that I have spoken" (Jn 12:49). On another occasion speaking about his actions he said, "Very truly I tell you, the Son can do nothing by himself; he can do only what he sees his Father doing, because whatever the Father does the Son also does" (Jn 5:19). These texts seem to imply that when his Father revealed

2   (New York: Oxford University Press, 1994), 280.

his will to him, Jesus had the unhesitating trust and confidence to believe that he had the God given authority and the power to carry it out, e.g., by means of healing.

The New Testament on the Faith of Jesus

Ian G. Wallis points out in his, *The Faith of Jesus Christ in Early Christian Traditions* that there is not one single, unambiguous reference to the faith of Jesus in the New Testament.[3] However, there are a number of ambiguous references which may imply that he did have faith. For instance, many translations of Heb 12:2 read, "look to Jesus the pioneer and perfecter of *our* faith." In Greek, the word "our" is not mentioned. The more accurate translation would be, "look to Jesus the pioneer and perfecter of faith." The phrase "perfecter of faith" could refer either to our faith in Jesus, the faith of Jesus himself, or possibly both together. If you read the story of the cure of the epileptic boy in Mk 9:17-29 you will find that the disciples were unable to liberate him because of their lack of faith. When the boy's father said that the demonic spirit, "has often cast him into the fire and into the water, to destroy him; but if you are able to do anything, have pity on us and help us," Jesus replied, "If you are able! – All things can be done for the *one* who believes." To whom does the word "one" refer? to the boy's father? to the disciples? or to Jesus himself? or to a combination of all three? When Jesus cast out the spirit, it was strongly implied that he was enabled to do so because he was the *one* who had exercised unwavering faith.

Did Jesus have the Charism of Faith?

If Jesus needed faith to exorcise the epileptic boy, and by extension to perform any healing or miracle, it would have been the charism rather than the other forms of faith that he had. It is mentioned in 1 Cor 12:9, "To some is given the charism of faith." It is the firm, expectant trust that is needed to perform deeds of power. Jesus

3   (Cambridge: Cambridge University Press, 1995).

described it very accurately when he said in Mk 11:23-24, "Have faith in God. I solemnly assure you, if you say to this mountain, 'Be taken up and thrown into the sea,' and if you do not doubt in your heart, but believe that what you say will come to pass, it will be done for you." Did Jesus have this kind of faith?

In view of what St Thomas said about Jesus not having the ordinary forms of faith, it may come as a surprise to know that he also said, "Christ is the first and chief teacher of spiritual doctrine and faith, according to Heb 2:3-4... Hence it is clear that *all* the gratuitous graces were most excellently in Christ as in the first and chief teacher of the faith."[4] That would strongly imply that Jesus had the charism of faith to move mountains (cf 1 Cor 12:9; 13:2). It is worth noting in this context that in par. 4 of his encyclical *On the Holy Spirit* (1897), Pope Leo XIII endorsed Thomas' view when he wrote, "In him (Christ)... were all the treasures of wisdom and knowledge, graces *gratis datae*, (i.e. charisms) virtues, and all other gifts foretold in the prophecies of Isaiah." So if we take Thomas' and Leo's words literally, it would seem that they were implying that Jesus exercised the charism of faith. This gift would have enabled him, among other things, to perform deeds of power such as healings, exorcisms and miracles.

Raising Lazarus as a Model of Faith?

It seems to me that we may have an outstanding example of the exercise of such faith, in the raising of Lazarus from the dead (Cf. Jn 11:1-45). To exercise the charism of faith a person firstly needs a revelation of God's will. We know that in all things Jesus was led by the Spirit. There is clear evidence that God the Father had made known to him that Lazarus would die and that he would be empowered to raise him from the dead. As a result Jesus was able to tell the apostles, in a prophetic manner, what was about to happen. When he got to the tomb of his beloved friend the people were

---

4   *Summa Theologiae*, third part, question 7, art. 7.

wailing and crying loudly in accordance with the Jewish custom of having intense mourning for four days. He was so moved, in an empathic way by the sadness of the mourners, that Jesus sighed and wept quietly.

Besides saying that he felt compassion, the Greek text implies that he was angry, not with the mourners, but with death and its ultimate master, the devil.[5] But he knew that it was God's will to reveal his glory by defeating the devil and raising Lazarus from the dead. What Jesus said to his Father at the tomb is really significant. "I thank you for hearing my prayer. I know indeed that you *always* hear me." It does sound like an expression of faith, of unhesitating confidence, that God will act in answer to a prayer which is in accord with his will. As he said to St Peter in Mk 11:24, "I tell you, whatever you ask for in prayer, believe that you have received it, and it will be yours."

If Jesus had this kind of faith, as I suspect he had, it was quite remarkable. By now, Lazarus was dead for four days. Jews believed that after the third day, the soul had definitely left the body. The corpse was already in a state of decay. So there is something utterly awe-inspiring and majestic about the words Jesus spoke, "Lazarus, here, come out!" As Is 55:11 promises, "my word... shall not return to me empty, but it shall accomplish that which I purpose, and succeed in the thing for which I sent it." The words of Jesus contained the power of their own fulfilment. As soon as they were uttered, the Holy Spirit, the Lord and giver of life, raised Lazarus from the dead. It was a mighty miracle, and as a result many of the people who witnessed it, believed in Jesus. It goes without saying that the raising of Lazarus prefigured Christ's own resurrection from the dead at the end of three days in the tomb.

---

5   Speaking of Jesus Heb 2:14 says, "Since therefore the children share in flesh and blood, he himself likewise partook of the same things, that through death he might destroy the one who has the power of death, that is, the devil."

Conclusion

It seems to me that the raising of Lazarus like other miracles of Jesus, indicates that as the Son of God, he is not only the object of our faith, in a qualified charismatic sense, he may also be our model of that faith. The implications are formidable. Because the biography of Jesus is our potential autobiography, he can enable us, when God wills it, to live in him the charism of faith which he exercised, by enabling us to occasionally heal the sick, drive out evil spirits, or if God so wills it, to perform miracles. We will explore this point in a little more depth in the next chapter.

CHAPTER FOUR

THE THINGS I DO, YOU WILL DO

In Jn 14:12-14 Jesus made an extraordinary promise to all those who believe in him, namely, "the things I do, you will do. "When one recalls what Jesus actually did, such as healing the sick, performing miracles, driving out evil spirits and raising the dead it is hard to believe that he literally meant what he said. As a result many commentators down the centuries interpreted his words to mean that we would evangelise in such a way as to bring about at least as many conversions as Jesus did, if not even more. Top scripture scholars such as Raymond Brown,[1] Rudolph Schnackenburg[2] and Francis J. Maloney[3] maintain, however, that such a reductionist interpretation does not do justice to what Jesus meant.[4] Yes his disciples would be empowered to evangelise effectively as Jesus did, but they would also be enabled to perform deeds of power as he did. The possibility of claiming the power of Christ's promise is rooted in our baptismal incorporation into his life.

Baptised into Christ

Thanks to baptism, Christians die to sin and are intimately united to Christ. Just as he was one with his Father, so, as a result of justification by grace through faith, we are made one with Christ. Our union with

---

1   *The Gospel According to John*, XIII-XXI, Anchor Bible, vol 29, part A (Yale: Anchor Bible 1970).

2   *Gospel According to St. John*, volume 2 (New York: The Seabury Press, 1982)

3   Sacra Pagina 4, *The Gospel of John* (Collegeville: The Liturgical Press, 1998)

4   Cf. Pat Collins, C.M., "Claiming the Promises of Scripture," in *Word and Spirit: Intimations of a New Springtime* (Dublin: Columba, 2011), 116-119.

Jesus is similar to his union with the Father. If we are going to do the same things as Jesus Christ, it is because we are united to him and he can act in and through us. Jesus himself talked about this, e.g., in his discourse on the vine and the branches. He said, "Remain in me, and I will remain in you. No branch can bear fruit by itself; it must remain in the vine. Neither can you bear fruit unless you remain in me" (Jn 15:4). Sometime later St. Paul testified in Gal 2:20, "I have been crucified with Christ and I no longer live, but Christ lives in me." While this is undoubtedly true from a theological and sacramental point of view since baptism, it may not necessarily be experientially true for every believer.[5] The baptism in the Holy Spirit which was mentioned in chapter one enables the truth about the presence and love of Jesus to fall the vital centimeters from head to heart, so that one can answer yes to Paul's question, "Do you not realize that Christ Jesus is in you" (2 Cor 13:5).

This awareness of intimate union with Jesus has profound implications. Implicit in this relationship is the realisation that the Christian community, as the body of Christ on earth, will have some members who will be able to heal the sick on Christ's behalf. As St Teresa of Avila once said, "Now Christ has no hands but yours." This truth is supported by the teaching of Paul in Phil 2:13 where he said, "God is at work in you, both to will and to work for his good pleasure." That verse makes three interrelated assertions which are well worth reflecting on in the context of healing ministry.

Firstly, St. Paul says, "God is at work in you." Christ is at work, not for us, or with us, but from *within* us through the action and gifts of the Holy Spirit. Secondly, St. Paul says that the Lord is at work within, enabling us to know and embrace the divine will, which sometimes includes healing. As he said in Col 1:9, "We continually ask God to fill you with the knowledge of his will through all the wisdom and understanding that the Spirit gives." This refers to practical rather than

---

5   There is an example of this paradox in Acts 8:14-17. Although the Samaritans had believed in the *kerygma* and had been baptised, the Spirit had not yet fallen on them in power until Peter and John prayed for them.

theoretical wisdom or knowledge. If you are in a situation where God wants you to heal, God can reveal the divine will. Thirdly, once the person intends to carry out God's will, he or she will be given the power, in their human weakness, to do so. St. Paul asserted that no matter how powerless a Christian may feel from a human point of view, "I can do everything (including healing) through him who gives me strength" (Phil 4:13). So once we hear the voice of the Lord, the Spirit will not only enable us to want to do God's will, it will also empower us to fulfil it.

Implications of the Divine Indwelling

St Paul's statement in Phil 2:13 found an echo in a treatise of St John Eudes (1601-1680), entitled, *The Life and the Kingdom of Jesus in Christian Souls*. He began by quoting a familiar verse from Col 1:24, "I rejoice in my sufferings for your sake, and in my flesh I complete what is lacking in Christ's afflictions for the sake of his body, that is, the church." Eudes believed that if Christians seek to continue and complete the suffering of Christ in their lives, surely that principle could be extended so as to apply to everything Jesus did, including healing. He wrote, "We can say that any true Christian, who is a member of Jesus Christ, and who is united to him by his grace, *continues* and *completes*, through all the actions that he carries out in the spirit of Christ, the actions that Jesus Christ accomplished during the time of his temporary life on earth."[6] The *Catechism of the Catholic Church* sums up the teaching of St John Eudes in par 521 where it says, "Christ enables us to live in him *all* that he himself lived, and he lives it in us."

This teaching was beautifully expressed in the following prayer of St. John Gabriel Perboyre, C.M. who was martyred in Wuhan, China in 1840, "O my Divine Saviour, transform me into yourself. May my hands be the hands of Jesus. May my tongue be the tongue of Jesus. Grant that every faculty of my body may serve only to glorify you. Above all, transform my soul and all its powers, so that my

---

6   The Classics of Western Spirituality, *Bérulle and the French School: Selected Writings* (New York: Paulist Press, 1989), 296.

memory, my will and my affections may be the memory, the will and the affections of Jesus. I pray you to destroy in me all that is not you. Grant that I may live but in you and for you, and that I may truly say with St. Paul, "I live, now not I, but Christ lives in me (Gal 2:20)." To grasp the implications of this prayer can open Christians up to the possibility of being able to pray effectively not only for healing or deliverance but even for miracles.

A story, which illustrates the foregoing points, describes how some American soldiers assisted French people in the aftermath of the D-day landings. In one town the locals asked the soldiers to help them to repair their church. As the pews and altar in the sanctuary were returned to their proper place, a statue of Jesus was found on the floor. His hands had been broken off and could not be found in the rubble. While they were trying to decide what to do about replacing Jesus' hands, the people placed the statue near the altar where it used to stand. Soon afterwards, the parishoners were deeply touched by what one of the soldiers had printed on a piece of paper and attached to the statue. It read, "From now on He has no hands, but yours."

Christ the healer dwells in the Christian Community

While, as the Son of God, Jesus exercised all the charisms himself, he does not give all his gifts to any one individual person. Rather he distributes them to his mystical body, i.e., the members of the Christian community. As Paul says in 1 Cor 12:8-10, "For to one is given through the Spirit the utterance of wisdom, and to another the utterance of knowledge according to the same Spirit, to another faith by the same Spirit, *to another gifts of healing* by the one Spirit, to another the working of miracles, to another prophecy, to another the ability to distinguish between spirits, to another various kinds of tongues, to another the interpretation of tongues." So if the spiritual seekers of our day are to experience God, they will find the Lord in and through the loving service and ministry of members of the Christian community, especially by means of deeds of power. As Paul said in 1 Cor 14:24-25, if, "an unbeliever or outsider enters, he is convicted by all, he is called to account by all, the secrets of his heart are disclosed, and so, falling on his face, he will worship God and declare that God is really among you."

Conclusion

This chapter has focused on two presences of Christ. Firstly, he is present in, and active through individual Christians. Secondly, the same Christ is present in and active through the Christian community. Rather than being opposing statements, they are complementary ones. It is precisely because Christ is present in individual persons that he is also present and active in and through the community. What obscures that sense of presence is unrepented sin in the life of individual Christians, and division in the life of the Christian community. As Ps 133:1; 3 says, "How wonderful, how beautiful, when brothers and sisters get along!... Yes, that's where God commands the blessing." That being so, it comes as no surprise that the devil's main counter strategy is to divide and thereby to conquer. Therefore there is a vital need for Christians to remain united. As St Paul said in Rm 14:19, "So then, let us aim for harmony in the Church and try to build each other up."

CHAPTER FIVE

....

SPIRITUAL HEALING

In chapter two we introduced the notion of spiritual healing within a holistic context which involved the interrelationship that exists in Christian thought between, soul, mind and body. At this point we are going to focus more specifically on the notion of spiritual healing. Once our soul, i.e., our innermost, animating self, is healed, it can in turn bring healing to the mind and body. In order to examine this topic we will have recourse to what some eminent psychologists have said about it as a result of their scientific observations. Before doing that, a cautionary note. In my book, *Mind and Spirit: Spirituality & Psychology in Dialogue*, I warned in a chapter entitled, "Psychology & Religion: An Uneasy Relationship" that the temptation to psychologise spirituality has to be avoided lest psychology becomes a *de facto* replacement for genuine Christian spirituality[1] which is often a characteristic of Gnostic forms of New Age Spirituality.[2] No doubt, psychology can throw light on spirituality, but it should not attempt to replace it. Three of the pioneers of 20th century psychology conducted an important discussion about the relationship between religious experience and mental health.

An important dispute

Freud was an atheist. In 1913 he wrote, "The analysis of individual human beings, teaches us in no uncertain terms that the god of each of them is formed in the likeness of his father, that his

---

1 (Dublin: Columba, 2006), 16-33.
2 Cf. Pat Collins, C.M., "New Age Spirituality" in *Spirituality for the 21ˢᵗ Century: Christian Living in a Secular Age* (Dublin: Columba, 1999), 106-113.

personal relation to God depends on his relation to his father in the flesh, and changes along with that relation. At bottom God is nothing other than an exalted father."[3] Freud regarded God as an illusion, based on the infantile need for a powerful father figure. Evidentially, Freud believed that religion was a form of universal, obsessional neurosis. So, if people wanted to become psychologically healthy, he maintained that they had to abandon their childish notion of God, take responsibility for their lives and learn to live with courage without the aid of this spiritual crutch.

Carl Jung came to the opposite conclusion. He said that unless people had spiritual experience they would be neurotic. He felt that the decline of religion in the modern era had, in fact, led to widespread neurosis. He wrote, "I am sure that everywhere the mental state of European man shows an alarming lack of balance. We are living undeniably in a period of the greatest restlessness, nervous tension, confusion, and disorientation of outlook."[4] Jung said that the human psyche could only be fulfilled if the self - his word for the soul[5] - enjoyed a conscious sense of the divine. In his book *Psychology & Western Religion* he wrote, "In thirty years I have treated many patients in the second half of life. Every one of them became ill because he or she had lost that which the living religions in every age have given their followers, (i.e. religious experience) and none of them was fully healed who did not regain his religious outlook."[6] Jung went on to add, "This of course has nothing whatever to do with a particular creed or membership of a church."[7] It is interesting to note that many of his patients

---

3   *Totem and Taboo,* (London: Routledge, 2015),171.
4   *Modern Man in Search of a Soul* (London: Routledge, 2005), 236.
5   Jung's understanding of the self is ambiguous. Speaking as a psychologist he said it referred to the unification of consciousness and unconsciousness in a person, and represented the psyche as a whole. But as someone who was open to religious experience, he felt that the self, was the locus of religious experience. I have long thought that there is confusion in Jung's psychology because he doesn't clearly differentiate between the soul and the self.
6   (London: Ark, 1988), 202.
7   Ibid., 202.

were practicing Christians, indeed some of them were clergymen. He argued that although they were committed to Christian doctrines and rituals, they got ill because, ironically, they were starved of conscious experience of God.

Viktor Frankl, a Jewish psychiatrist was imprisoned in a number of concentration camps, during World War II. He noticed that, all things being equal, some prisoners were better able to survive than others. He discovered that it was the prisoners who had a sense of unconditional meaning who could endure great hardship, whereas, those who hadn't such a sense of meaning, often lost the will to live and died as a result of such things as disease or suicide. Consequently, Frankl tried to introduce into psychotherapy a point of view that saw in human existence not only a Freudian *will to pleasure*, an Adlerian *will to power*, a Jungian will to *individuation*, or a Maslonian will to *self-actualization*, what he referred to as the *will to meaning*. He recounted, "Perhaps the deepest experience which I myself had in the concentration camp was that, while the concern of most people was summed up by the question, 'Will we survive the camp?' - for if not, then this suffering has no sense - the question which in contrast beset me was, 'has this whole suffering, this dying a meaning?' - for if not, then ultimately there is no sense in surviving. For a life whose meaning stands or falls upon whether one survives or not, a life, that is, whose meaning depends upon such a happenstance, such a life would not really be worth living at all."[8]

Contrary to Freud's position which approved of the fact that in modern culture the religious sense is often ignored, Frankl believed that the consequent lack of meaning leads people to suffer from a vacuum, an emptiness at the centre of their lives, what he called "existential frustration." It can lead to boredom, depression, *ennui* and neurosis. He felt that if people suppressed the spiritual sense, they would end up in a kind of idolatry by making things like pleasure, power, and popularity into unsatisfactory substitutes for

8   *Man's Search for Meaning* (New York: Pocket Books, 1963), 183.

absolute meaning.[9] He maintained that this existential vacuum can also result in addictions or suicide. In other words when the human spirit is deprived of the oxygen of meaning the person becomes psychologically unbalanced and self-destructive.

Empirical Research

In an article entitled "Religious Orientation and Psychological Well-being: The Role of the Frequency of Personal Prayer," which was published in *The British Journal of Health Psychology* (1999), three researchers examined the effects of what Gordon Allport referred to as 'intrinsic religion' on mental health.[10] People who have intrinsic, as opposed to extrinsic religion, are those who have internalised their faith in such a way that it influences every aspect of their everyday lives. Instead of engaging in infrequent prayer of a formal, impersonal, self-centred kind, they spend time in regular periods of prayer of a personal, God-centred kind. Instead of primarily seeking to know what God can do for them, they seek to know what they can do for God. Consequently, they are not only more inclined to have a conscious awareness of the divine, they are also more likely to have higher self-esteem together with lower levels of anxiety and depression.

Dr Patricia Casey, a professor of psychiatry in University College Dublin is the author of *The Psycho-social Benefits of Religious Practice*, which was published by the Iona Institute in 2008. She has said, "the overwhelming weight of evidence so far is that being actively engaged in religious participation is psychologically beneficial for individuals, and also carries a range of social benefits relating to everything from marital stability to crime and to suicide."[11] The booklet examines various scientific studies conducted in this area which show that religious practice is associated, on average, with

9   *Man's Search for Meaning*, op. cit., 170.
10   Allport, G. W., & Ross, J. M. (1967). "Personal religious orientation and prejudice" in *Journal of Personality and Social Psychology*, 5(4), 432–443.
11   (Dublin: Iona Institute, 2009), 35.

lower levels of, depression; of marital breakdown; of alcohol and drug abuse; of pregnancy among teenagers; faster recovery from bereavement and illness; together with longer life expectancy, etc. While Dr Casey focused on religious practice, I think that her booklet would have been even more helpful if it had focused more on religious experience.

Dr. Harold G. Koenig, is a psychiatrist on the faculty of Duke University, USA. As a result of his research, he says, like Professor Casey that, all things being equal, people who measure higher on religion/spirituality variables typically have improved mental and physical health. In a book entitled *Spirituality and Religion Within the Culture of Medicine: From Evidence to Practice* he states, "Much research has now been published on relationships between religion, spirituality and health in older adults. The vast majority of that research suggests that religious or spiritual involvement is associated with better mental, social, behavioural and physical health."[12]

Bill Wilson, was one of the founders of Alcoholics Anonymous. An acquaintance of his, Roland Hazard, travelled to Switzerland to get psychological help for his alcoholism from Carl Jung. However, he relapsed following his therapy and decided to return. Jung stated there was nothing more that psychiatry or medicine could do for him. There was just one remaining hope. Jung said that, occasionally alcoholics could recover from their debilitating addiction as a result of experiencing religious conversion. So Hazard attended meetings of the Oxford Group, a Christian evangelical movement active in Europe. He experienced a spiritual awakening and never drank again.

When Bill Wilson, a chronic alcoholic himself, heard from a friend called Edwin Thacher about Hazard's recovery, he began to long for a similar religious awakening. He described how his desire gave way to fulfilment, "Suddenly my room blazed with an indescribable white light. I was seized with an ecstasy beyond description... Then, seen in the mind's eye, there was a mountain.

---

12 (New York: Oxford University Press, 2017), 109-128.

I stood upon its summit, where a great wind blew. A wind, not of air, but of spirit. In great, clean strength, it blew right through me. Then came the blazing thought, "You are a free man"... a great peace stole over me... seemed to be possessed by the absolute, and the curious conviction deepened that no matter how wrong things seemed to be, there could be no question of the ultimate rightness of God's universe. For the first time I felt I really belonged."[13] Having experienced the Higher Power, Wilson never drank again. Years later Jung stated in a letter to Wilson, "alcohol" in Latin is *spiritus*, and you use the same word for the highest religious experience as well as for the most depraving poison. The helpful formula therefore is: *spiritus contra spiritum* (i.e. spirit against spirit). "As a deer pants for flowing streams, so pants my soul for you, O God" (Ps 42:1)."[14]

Conclusion

I'm convinced that there are many people in modern society who are suffering from psychological and behavioural problems that are spiritual in origin. Like Bill Wilson, they need a spiritual awakening in the form of baptism in the Spirit, in order to aid their recovery. It can lead to a therapeutic effect. Once the soul, the innermost self, is locked on to ultimate meaning, once the person has an unshakable faith conviction of being loved in an unconditional way by Jesus, the person's mind and body can develop in a more healthy, holistic way. He or she develops an inner awareness that God is guiding the world, and a conviction that life can be lived in accord with divine providence so that one is no longer being tossed about on a chaotic sea of relativism.

---

13 Dick B, *The Conversion of Bill W: More on the Creator's Role in Early AA* (Kihi: Paradise Research Publications, 2006), 134-135.

14 *The Grapevine*, International Monthly Journal of Alcoholics Anonymous, Vol. 24, No. 8, Jan 1968. See also Pat Collins, C.M., "Freedom From Addiction," in *Freedom From Evil Spirits: Released from Fear, Addiction and the Devil* (Dublin: Columba, 2019), 77-124.

CHAPTER SIX

....

DELIVERANCE &
SPIRITUAL HEALING

The previous chapter introduced the subject of spiritual healing as a result of genuine religious experience which can have therapeutic knock-on effects on mind and body. The New Testament stresses the fact that the enemy of our souls has great influence in the world. In Rev 12:9 we read that, "Satan,... was hurled to the earth, and his angels with him." So his main sphere of influence is right here in our world. Jesus variously referred to the devil as, "the ruler" and "the prince" of this world (Jn 12:31; 14:30; 16:11). St Paul went so far as to refer to him as, "the god of this world" (2 Cor 4:4). St John observed that, "the whole world lies in the power of the evil one" (1 Jn 5:19). In other words, while the evil influence of the devil is often not recognised or acknowledged, it is nevertheless pervasive and malevolent, afflicting people in soul, mind and body. As a result, there is a growing need in Western countries for the ministry of deliverance.

Deliverance in Christian thought

Recently I read that in August 2019 Fr. Arturo Sosa, the Superior General, of the Jesuits, said that, in his opinion, the devil is merely a symbol of evil, but not a supernatural person. Though he espouses a liberal point of view that is common in Christian circles, it is not orthodox. Pope Francis, a Jesuit himself, endorsed the Biblical point of view when he said in par. 161 of *Rejoice and be Glad*, "we should not think of the devil as a myth, a representation, a symbol, a figure of speech or an idea." He has pointed out in par. 160 that the words, "deliver us from evil" do not refer to evil in the abstract but to Satan the evil one, a personal being who assails us."[1] So, in the final petition of the Lord's Prayer, Jesus teaches us to ask to be delivered from the temptations, illusions, and false inspirations of the devil who wanders through the world, sometimes masquerading as an angel of light, (cf. 2 Cor 11:14), seeking the ruin of souls.

The New Testament tells us how to protect ourselves from the wiles of the Devil. St Peter counselled, "*Stay alert! Watch out* for your great enemy, the devil. He prowls around like a roaring lion, looking for someone to devour. *Resist him, steadfast in faith*" (1 Pt 5:8). St James added, "*humble* yourselves before God. *Resist* the devil, and he will flee from you" (Jm 4:7). Take note of the verbs in these verses. Rather than being words of advice, the phrases such as "stay alert," "be humble" and "resist the devil firm in faith" are words of command. Rely on God's Spirit, at work within you, and the Spirit will enable you to obey them. St Paul tells us in Eph 6:16 that, "The shield of faith puts out *all* the fiery darts of the evil one." Scripture repeatedly makes it clear that the Lord is our spiritual shield. For example, in Prov 30:5 we read, "He (God) is a shield to those who take refuge in him" and in Ps 144:2, "He is my loving God, my fortress, my stronghold and my deliverer, my shield in whom I take refuge." When you feel under attack from evil, raise your shield by saying, "Jesus I trust in you." Nestle through faith in Christ, don't wrestle with the evil one.

Sad to say, many people ignore this advice. They resemble the Jews of old who were mentioned in Judges 21:25, "In those days Israel had no king; all the people did whatever seemed right in their own eyes." As a result of lacking a moral compass, many people live in a permissive way, grievous sins are committed, mental health deteriorates, inappropriate activity increases, the social media fill with hateful and untruthful postings, and problems with

---

1   See Pope Francis, *Rebuking the Devil* (Washington: United States Conference of Catholic Bishops, 2019), 9.

addiction multiply. Why is it that so many people seem to succumb knowingly or unwittingly to the temptations, illusions and false inspirations of the evil one?

Here are some of common causes. Pope Pius XII said it was often due to a denial of the devil's very existence. Un-repented sin, of a serious kind, is another common entry point, as is the influence of ancestral spirits and curses. Traumatic experiences associated with unresolved negative feelings is another gateway, as are unforgiveness and resentment; addictions to things like drink, drugs and pornography; involvement in occult activities such as palmistry, spiritualism, Reiki, kundalini, fortune telling, witchcraft, contacting the dead, consulting mediums, channelling, religious forms of yoga, and using a Ouija board or tarot cards in a misguided effort to contact the world of spirits or to gain control over their lives and their futures. By engaging in these and similar New Age activities, people can unwittingly break the first commandment. Finally, there can be ungodly soul ties in a person's life as a result of illicit sexual relationships and practices, which may have involved extra marital promises, commitments and agreements.[2]

As a result of the devil getting a foothold the following problems can ensue

1) *Oppression*, i.e., when evil spirits attack a person's exterior life and influence his or her bodily health, finances, work situation, family and other relationships;

2) *Obsession*, i.e., when the evil spirits impinge on part of the personality. It can result in disturbing, obsessive thoughts planted by the enemy who may cause nightmares. The afflicted person may hear inner voices urging them, for instance, to commit acts of violence or self harm.

3) *Possession*, i.e., when a person's whole inner life seems to be subject to the influence of the devil. According to the

---

2   For a more extended treatment of this topic see Pat Collins, C.M., "Freedom From Oppressive Evil Spirits" in *Freedom From Evil Spirits: Released From Fear, Addiction and the Devil* (Dublin: Columba, 2019), 155-159.

Vatican guidelines issued in 1999, "the person who claims to be possessed must be evaluated by doctors to rule out a mental or physical illness."

In his book, *Deliverance from Evil Spirits: A Practical Manual*, the late Francis McNutt listed four main kinds of spirits that can be involved once they get a foothold, spirits of the occult; spirits of sin; spirits of trauma; and ancestral spirits, i.e., either demons masquerading as dead people, or souls of the dead who need rest.[3]

Unbound

If any of these spirits are afflicting a Christian's soul how can he or she experience deliverance and healing? Neal Lozano, an American Catholic layman has developed a very helpful method involving five keys which he has described in his book *Unbound*.[4] An oppressed individual could help him or herself by using the keys. What is more common however, is that the afflicted person is helped to apply the keys with the assistance of one or two other trained Christians. They begin by trying to identify, in a diagnostic way, how the evil one was given an opportunity to get a foothold in people's lives. Then they focus on the five keys that open the door to liberation.

Firstly, they are asked to *repent* of any way they gave the devil a foothold in their life. Catholics can do this by receiving the sacrament of reconciliation. Secondly, they are urged, with God's help, to *forgive* anyone who played a part in their vulnerability to spiritual oppression. Thirdly, they are encouraged to *renounce* any false ideas they have about themselves or God, e.g., "I'm unlovable," "my life isn't worth living" or "God is remote, detached and demanding" etc. They also renounce whatever spirit is oppressing them such as a lustful, occult, violent or blasphemous spirit. Fourthly, they tell

---

3   (London: Hodder & Stoughton, 1996), 90-97.
4   Lozano, Neal. *Unbound: A Practical Guide to Deliverance*. (Grand Rapids, Michigan: Chosen, 2003).

afflicted people to *command* the spirit to leave them in the name of the Lord Jesus. They are encouraged to do this in a wholehearted way with expectant faith. Fifthly, they ask people to call down God the Father's *blessing* upon themselves, to fill and protect them from the Evil One. I have found that it can be very helpful at this stage to get people who want to be unbound to say the so-called Miracle Prayer, which reads as follows.

> "Lord Jesus, I come before you, just as I am. I am sorry for my sins, I repent of them, please forgive me. In your Name, I forgive all others for what they have done against me. I renounce Satan, the evil spirits and all their works. I give my entire self, to you Lord Jesus. I accept you as my Lord and Saviour. Heal me, change me, strengthen me in body, soul, and spirit. Come Lord Jesus, cover me with your precious blood, and fill me with your Holy Spirit. I love you Lord Jesus. I praise you Lord Jesus. I thank you Jesus, I shall follow you every day for the rest of my life. Amen."

To pray for deliverance is to form a caring relationship with people. It is important therefore that, afterwards, one keeps in touch with them in order to see how they are getting on and whether they may need further ministry. It is also important to encourage those who were formerly afflicted to strengthen their spiritual lives, e.g., by means of daily prayer; reading of scripture, reception of the sacraments, resisting temptation to sin, etc. The closer they come to God, the more they will be able to ward off demonic influences. Finally, it is important to note that only a priest appointed by a bishop can perform a solemn exorcism for someone who is possessed. In my experience that pastoral need rarely arises.[5]

---

5   Cf. *The Code of Canon Law*, canon 1172.

Conclusion

Following effective prayer for deliverance, many of those who have been released from the influence of evil spirits will still have inner hurts which will need to be healed by means of such normal things as psychotherapy, counselling and prayer for healing of memories. I have found, that until spiritual oppression is discerned and lifted, the therapeutic activities already mentioned will not be very effective. That said, when people are liberated from the influence of evil spirits, they will often experience an improvement in their mental and physical health.

Finally, while it would not be true to say that the devil directly causes all sickness, it would be theologically true to say that he has an indirect influence due to the fact that, as a result of tempting Adam and Eve to disobey God, suffering and death came into the world. It would also be true to say that, in some cases in the New Testament, there is a clear link between an illness, disease or handicap and the activity of the evil one. Jesus made those distinctions. In Mt 9:32-33, for example, we are told that a man who was demon-possessed and could not speak was brought to Jesus. And when the demon was driven out, the man who had been mute began to speak. The crowd was amazed and said, "Nothing like this has ever been seen in Israel." In Acts 10:38 St Peter testified that Jesus, "went about doing good, and healing all that were oppressed by the devil; for God was with him." Nowadays spiritual discernment is needed in order to diagnose what is really involved when people ask for healing prayer. In a minority of cases, where there may be a diabolical dimension, deliverance prayer may be needed as part of the healing process. It seems clear from the ministry of Smith Wigglesworth, that he often engaged in this kind of discernment and ministered with a combination of deliverance and healing prayer with considerable success.

CHAPTER SEVEN

....

INNER HEALING

Meister Eckhart (1260-1327 A.D.) a well known Dominican wrote these words, "If you love yourself, you love everybody else as you do yourself. As long as you love another person less than you love yourself, you will not succeed in loving yourself; but if you love all alike, including yourself, you will love them as one person and that person is both God and man. Thus he is a great and righteous person who, loving himself, loves all others equally."[1] In modern terms one could say that healthy minded people are those who *accept themselves* as they are, warts and all; who *are themselves* without wearing a mask or acting a part; and who *forget themselves* in outgoing, empathic love for others. The inability to love others in this way is often due to the fact that many people are suffering from unacknowledged and unresolved inner hurts and pain.

Neurosis

If the truth be told many people are neurotic to a greater or lesser extent. "Neurosis is an inner cleavage," wrote Carl Jung, "the state of being at war with oneself. Everything that accentuates this cleavage makes the patient worse, and everything that mitigates it tends to heal him. What drives people to war with themselves is the suspicion that they consist of two persons in opposition to one another. The conflict may be between the sensual and the spiritual, between the ego and the shadow... Neurosis is a splitting of personality."[2] In spite of talking about many different presenting problems, those who ask for prayer

---

1   Quoted by Erich Fromm in *The Art of Loving: An Inquiry Into the Nature of Love* (New York: Harper and Brothers, 1956), 58.
2   "Psychotherapists or the Clergy" in *Psychology and Western Religion* (London: Ark, 1988), 208-209.

for inner healing will often be suffering from the same root problem, namely a splitting of the personality between the acceptable and the lovable side from the part that is rejected, and unlovable. The story of Dr Jekyll and Mr Hyde was Robert Louis Stevenson's memorable way of illustrating this form of inner alienation.

The importance of self-acceptance

Speaking about inner alienation Jung wrote these striking words in his book *Modern Man in Search of a Soul,* "Perhaps this sounds very simple, but simple things are always the most difficult. In real life it requires the greatest discipline to be simple, and the acceptance of oneself is the essence of the moral problem and the epitome of a whole outlook upon life. That I feed the hungry, forgive an insult and love my enemy in the name of Christ – all these are undoubtedly great virtues ... After all, what I do for the least of my brothers and sisters, that I do to Christ. But what if I discover that the least among them all, the poorest of all the beggars, the worst of all the offenders, the very enemy himself – that these are within me, and that I stand in need of the handout of my own kindness – that I myself am the enemy who must be loved – what then?"[3] This quotation throws an interesting light on what Jesus might have meant when he said, "Love your neighbour as yourself" (Mk 12:31).

Low self-esteem

People with poor self-acceptance, and that is most of us, often suffer from low self-esteem. It is a common experience which is mainly due to shortcomings in the care and nurturing of children. Here are some of the predictable signs of low self-esteem which I have dealt with more fully elsewhere.[4]

- Lack of self-confidence and shyness.
- Difficulties in trusting others or sharing one's most intimate thoughts, feelings and memories with them. Deep down

---

3   *Psychology and Western Religion,* op. cit., 207.
4   Cf. Pat Collins, C.M., "Self-esteem and the Love of God," in *Growing in Health and Grace* (Galway: Campus, 1991), 27-43.

they feel, if people knew me as I really am, they would dislike me as much as I already dislike and reject my inferior self.

- Difficulties in accepting gratitude or praise.
- Difficulties in asking for, or accepting help from others.
- An exaggerated fear of failure, often associated with a compensatory tendency to brag.
- Feelings of jealousy and envy which are rooted in insecurity in relationships.
- Sexual difficulties of all kinds which are often rooted in negative feelings rather than lust.
- Co-dependency and addictions of all kinds such as substance abuse, e.g., alcoholism; and process addictions, e.g., compulsive shopping or gambling.
- A tendency to judge and condemn others in a harsh way, i.e., seeing the speck in the neighbour's eye while overlooking the log in one's own (cf. Mt 7:3-5).
- Over sensitivity so that one is not only easily hurt but also prone to react emotionally in a negative and defensive way.
- A tendency to self-absorption, excessive self-reference and a lack of empathy.
- Unhealthy levels of emotional and physical stress.

The experience of hurtful trauma

All of us can be traumatised by "the slings and arrows of outrageous fortune."[5] Unfortunately bad things can, and do, happen to good people. Often, they suffer at the hands of others, as for example, when men and women are robbed, beaten up, or ruthlessly exploited or experience an accident or a natural disaster. Some young people are traumatised by witnessing violence in the home, e.g., children seeing their angry and drunken father beating up their mother. Others are badly affected by such things as betrayal, or finding the corpse of someone who committed suicide by hanging.

---

5   William Shakespeare, *Hamlet*, Act III, Scene 1, line 1751.

While the list of potential hurts is almost endless, the effects are often similar.

Clearly, many, if not most people are wounded psychologically & emotionally. In the more extreme cases of hurt, such as is the case in the aftermath of child sex abuse, the pain is so bad that the person may completely repress the memory and its associated negative feelings in the unconscious. Rather than going away they exert a malign, but unrecognized influence upon the person's emotional attitudes, perceptions and reactions to the events of life. Here are a few examples.

1) Often these repressed feelings are a cause of stress which leaves the body more vulnerable to sickness and infection. In other words, as was noted in chapter two, negative feelings can be displaced, in a psychosomatic way, into unhealthy physical states.

2) Repressed hurts can also exert a negative influence on conscious attitudes, feelings and behaviours such as phobias, irrational anger and a tendency to self-harm, suicidal tendencies and addictions.

3) Needless to say relationships suffer, because unconscious feelings of a negative kind keep on undermining a conscious sense of connection. For example, a woman who has repressed the memory of being raped as a young woman may be physically frigid in spite of the fact that she loves her husband deeply. A person suffering from separation anxiety may be lonely because he or she finds it very difficult to trust anyone enough to reveal their true self to them. As a result they never feel loved as they really are, lack spontaneity, and identify with their persona, i.e., the personality that an individual projects to others, as differentiated from his or her authentic self.

4) Depression and anxiety states are also common because anger associated with psychic traumas is often repressed, for one reason or another. This is the subject of the next chapter. As a result it can attack the person and manifest itself,

firstly in the form of anxiety, and later on as reactive depression. In other cases, memory of a trauma is not completely repressed. But, for one reason or another, the unfortunate victim is unable to cope with the consequences, e.g., post traumatic stress disorder and passive aggressive behaviour.

Over the years, I have found that the extent to which parents fail to transform their own inner pain, as a result of their personal life hurts, is the extent to which they will tend to transmit it to their children. As a result, their offspring will tend to absorb the distorted attitudes of their parents or carers, such as perfectionism and anxiety, in an unconscious way. As a result there are not adequate or proportionate explanations in their own life stories to account for the emotional problems they have to cope with. In reality, one or other of their parents may have passed on the baton of dysfunctionality to their offspring (cf. Deut 5:9).

Indeed, some psychologists would argue that traumas that went unresolved in previous generations of a family may continue to exert a negative, but unacknowledged influence on members of the present generation. With this in mind, Christian psychiatrist, Dr. Kenneth McAll introduced the practice of healing the family tree, by praying for release from the effects of inherited ancestral wounds.[6] I can remember spending many hours in conversation with Doctor McAll in the 1980s. He believed that problems such as an eating disorder, might have its root cause in the unresolved problems of deceased relatives. Although he was a Presbyterian, he told me that he felt that one possible cure was to offer a requiem mass for the restless dead. In Catholic circles, that view has given rise to, "healing the family tree" Masses. I can recall celebrating such a Mass for intergenerational healing at the request of a family I knew in Dublin one of whose members suffered from an eating disorder. When we reached the offertory a family member put a list

6   *Healing the Family Tree* (London: SPCK, 2013).

of deceased relatives on the altar. We prayed that God would have mercy on them, that they would rest in peace, and that all negative ties between them and the living would be severed. Immediately afterwards a daughter who had been suffering from anorexia nervosa for many years recovered completely.

The Experience of Anxiety

Psychologists say that although fear and anxiety are interconnected they are different. Whereas fear has a particular object, whether real or imaginary, e.g., possible loss of one's job, anxiety has no particular focus. It is a fear about everything in general and nothing in particular. Anxiety has ontological and psychological roots. As finite, contingent creatures we are not the adequate explanation of our own existence which is threatened by the prospect of falling back, at the time of our death, into the darkness of the uncreated night from which we came. From a psychological point of view, anxiety has many roots, but in my experience one important one is, what is known, as separation anxiety which often dates back to early childhood. That topic will be briefly dealt with in the chapters on the father and the mother wound. For many years St Therese of Lisieux suffered greatly from chronic anxiety as a result of being parted for a time from her mother shortly after her birth. It is significant that she began to be healed of her anxiety at the age of fourteen when she experienced a revelation of God's great love for her, at a Christmas Eve Mass, in 1886. Evidently, baptism in the Spirit was a great antidote to her anxious fear. As scripture says, "There is no fear in love. But perfect love drives out fear, because fear has to do with punishment" (1 Jn 4:18). I have written at greater length about the topic of anxious fear and how to overcome it in the first section of *Freedom From Evil Spirits*.[7]

---

7   (Dublin: Columba, 2019), 21-73.

Conclusion

The subject of inner healing is a large and complex one to which we will return in later chapters. Those who need such healing are well advised to try to acknowledge their need, and as much as possible, its causes. One can pray to the Lord for such self-awareness of hurting memories and their associated negative feelings. Carl Jung wrote, "Real liberation comes not from glossing over or repressing painful states of feeling, but only from experiencing them to the full."[8] The Holy Spirit can help in doing this. As the psalmist wrote, "Search me, God, and know my heart; test me and know my anxious thoughts. See if there is any offensive way in me, and lead me in the way everlasting" (Ps 139:23-24). There is something sacred about inner woundedness, because it can become the birthplace of great blessing due to the fact that the Holy Spirit, the Paraclete, is God's answer to the cry of the broken human heart. As Ps 34:18 says, "The Lord is close to the broken hearted and saves/heals those who are crushed in spirit."

---

8   *The Archetypes and the Collective Unconscious*, CW 9i, para. 587

CHAPTER EIGHT

....

RELIEVING DEPRESSION

According to the World Health Organisation depression, the "blue plague" is a common illness, with an estimated 264 million people affected worldwide. As someone who is not a mental health professional I have noticed over the years that there are different kinds of depression such as:

- Endogenous, which is largely due to changes in the electrochemical activity of the brain which may have an inherited cause.

- Seasonal affective disorder, a kind of depression which can recur each Winter when there is a lack of sunlight, hence the term, "The Winter blues."

- Bi-polar disorder, which can involve mood swings that go from elation to depression. It probably has a biological and genetic root.

- Post-natal depression, experienced by 10 to 15% of mothers in the year after giving birth.

- Reactive depression, is a mood disorder triggered by a specific event/s of a stressful nature. This could be anything that changes or threatens to change a person's everyday routine or expectations. It can be triggered by such things as the death of a loved one, the end of a relationship, loss of a job, a car accident, or some kind of rejection etc.

This chapter will focus on some aspects of reactive type depressions because they are quite common. Each one of us has physical, psychological and spiritual needs. Psychologist *Roberto Assagioli* (1888-1974) has suggested that there are six of them; to preserve life; sexual intimacy; security; affirmation, knowledge; and meaning. Abraham Maslow (1908-1970), said there were five basic needs; physical; safety; love; esteem; and self-actualization. When needs like these are satisfied we feel happy and fulfilled. When they are denied by people, circumstances or events we feel a sense of deprivation, loss and hurt. It is this sense of missing out that gives rise to a defensive feeling of anger. As Francis Bacon wrote in one of his *Essays*, "no man is angry that feels not himself hurt."[1] Anger can be turned inward against oneself in a damaging way.

There are some typical triggers for reactive depression which cause a sense of deprivation, hurt and loss. There can be the break-up of a romantic relationship; marital problems ending in divorce; having a baby perhaps with a handicap; negative financial situations, e.g., debt or losing a job; the death of a loved one, perhaps as a result of suicide; social issues at school or work, e.g., being bullied; life-or-death experiences such as physical assault, a car crash; a natural disaster; serious medical illness or handicap; having a so-called neighbour from hell living next door. Not only are situations and events like these, stressful, they can evoke feelings of impotence, helplessness, hopelessness, sadness and a good deal of anger against fate, people and God.

Many people were reared in homes where anger was not acceptable for one reason or another. So children learned to suppress their anger in order to retain the affection and approval of their parents. As this kind of denial and repression was repeated it became second nature. By the time they reached adulthood some of these people found it very hard to acknowledge any anger. They would have the *emotion* stored in their bodies, like energy stored in a battery, which would cause such things as headaches, fibromyalgia and shortness of breath, but without experiencing any *feeling* of anger. Anger which has been repressed and over a period of time, typically mutates into feelings of anxiety, inadequacy, insecurity and

1   *The Philosophical Works of Francis Bacon* in *Essays,* LVII (New York: Routledge, 1905), 804.

even panic. If the repressed anger is strong and persistent, but unacknowledged, it can turn into depression. So it is my belief that, while quite often depression is the presenting problem, the root cause is negative feeling, including anger which has been buried alive in the unconscious mind.

Getting in touch with repressed feelings

If there is truth in the dynamic just described, then a depressed person's healing begins by (a) *recovering* repressed feelings of a negative kind and recalling the painful events that evoked them; (b) *naming* those feelings, (c) *owning* them in a heartfelt way; (d) *understanding* them; and (e) *expressing* them. It has to be acknowledged at this point that some people get so depressed that they are incapable of talking about the foregoing points. The only thing that helps them at times like that, besides prayer ministry, is to take prescribed antidepressants, until such a time as they are capable of talking about the roots of their problem. While these five steps are helpful when helping clients to get in touch with their memories and any associated feelings, we will use them here to focus principally on repressed anger.

A] Recovering repressed feelings.

Begin by asking the Lord to search you and to know you so that you get in touch with the truth of your own heart. Then take notice of your physical state. Is your mouth dry? Are your muscles aching? Have you a headache? Are you perspiring? Communicate with your body, asking it to translate its emotional states into conscious feelings together with their associated memories. This usually happens by means of spontaneously generated images, e.g., remembering a feeling laden incident seen on T.V. Your unconscious mind might have suggested that image because it evokes a feeling to do with your past which you find hard to acknowledge. In this connection it is worth recalling any dreams you may have had. As Freud said, they are "the royal road to the unconscious,"[2] i.e., to repressed feelings and memories. When you recall a dream ask yourself, what was the main feeling it contained? That may remind you of an unacknowledged feeling during the previous forty eight hours. What evoked it? Could it be an echo of a similar reaction in your past life? Ask yourself whether you can remember a hurtful memory which may have evoked your negative feeling many years ago.

B] Name your feelings.
Many of us, especially men, can be fairly inarticulate when it comes to feelings. Try to name how you feel by going beyond vague generalities such as, "good" or "bad," to be more specific, e.g., "I felt angry, let down, violated."

C] Own your feelings.
Sometimes we keep our feelings at arm's length. Do you acknowledge in a detached sort of way that, "I have anger, a feeling of being let down or violated" instead of owning the feeling in a heartfelt way by saying, "I am angry, I have been let down and violated."

D] Understand your feelings
What unfulfilled need, expectation, perception, value or belief evoked your feelings? What in your earlier life might have conditioned the way you look at things? Is your way of perceiving things really realistic and in accord with your professed Christian beliefs and values?

E] Express your feelings
There is an educational adage which states that "there is nothing impressed which is not expressed." You can express your feelings in a number of ways, by journaling, expressing them to a counsellor, friend or healer, to God in prayer.

2   *The Interpretation of Dreams* (1900), from *The Standard Edition of the Complete Psychological Works of Sigmund Freud*, translated by James Strachey.

A number of years ago I heard someone say, "Although other people can evoke our feelings, including anger, the causes lie within." So there is no point in blaming others and saying, "You caused me to be angry!" Anger is the responsibility of those who experience it. It is rooted in a person's unique expectations, values, beliefs, and perceptions. Some will be unrealistic, e.g., everyone should love me. Others will be questionable, e.g. a married man feels rejected, humiliated and angry when a single woman fails to respond to his flirtatious behaviour. Some anger is due to misinterpretation, e.g., a lonely man who is seeking a relationship, may easily misunderstand the responses of a charming woman to mean that she is offering more than just a casual friendship. When his hopes turn to disappointment he may feel rejected and angry. While the woman's response may have evoked his anger the cause lies in his inaccurate perception. When a depressed person asks a healer for help, the latter can often use this five stage approach to assist the depressed person to get in touch with the causes of his or her despondency and dejection.

Forgiveness and depression

When I was involved in conducting parish missions around Ireland, I used to meet with people who were very seriously depressed, some of them for many years, despite the best efforts of doctors and psychiatrists to help them. I had a woman friend, who had a wonderful gift of healing, especially depressive states. I can remember sending two women to see her at different times, one from Newry, the other from Dublin. My friend talked to each of them, tried to get to the root cause of their depression and then she prayed for them. Although they had endured inner darkness for many years both women were completely healed. When I asked her what she had done that was so obviously effective, she offered a very simple answer.

Firstly, she talked about the compassion that was evoked within her as she listened to the women's sad stories. They brought tears to her eyes, and she said, that she sensed how much the Lord loved them and how he wanted to help them. I know it sounds simplistic, but heartfelt love is the key to healing, there is no technique or effort that can replace it.[3]

Secondly, in both cases my friend found that the women were angry and resentful about things which were either done or left undone in their pasts. She said that she invited each woman to offer forgiveness to those who had caused them pain while leading both in a sincere prayer of forgiveness. Then my friend prayed that the Lord, by his Holy Spirit, would bring them healing, light and peace. In both cases, her prayer was heard in a remarkable way, but she stressed the fact that forgiveness was the key to their inner healing.

Expressing anger to God

Some of the people who are depressed will sometimes have an unconscious feeling of anger against God, in the belief that the Lord has failed to protect or save them from hurt and loss. That repressed anger/rage and resentment needs to be acknowledged and expressed to God. Otherwise, it can not only block a person's sense of conscious relationship with the Lord, it can also lead to depression. In order to be healed of the depression, therefore, it is important to acknowledge the anger and to express it without censorship to the Lord. I can remember reading a powerful example of that kind of dynamic in Dr Frank Lake's book, *With Respect: A Doctor's Response to a Healing Pope.* A depressed woman who he had tried to help during a retreat told him how she overcame her illness.

> "I went alone into the chapel. The panic of what I would do to myself to stop the intolerable pain drove me to

---

3   There are many forms of psychotherapy which are the outcomes of different psychological theories. Research indicates that, in spite of their theoretical differences, all of them can be efficacious if the therapist has empathy for the client. Cf. Carr, G.D. (2011). "Psychotherapy research: Implications for practice," in *Psychiatric Times*, 28.8, 31.

my knees, my tongue moving incoherently, my soul stretched tight with a weeping longing. When I was still left alone my very despair drove me to a horror and fury which was unafraid of recrimination. I was staggered by the milk-and-water apologetic God who could not calm this storm, who smiled sympathetically but abstractly and whom I could not touch. We can bear humans to fall off their pedestals but not God himself. After the first stunning realisation of who God was, my whole mind, soul and body came into co-ordination and rose in unity to hate with entire, full-blooded, no holds barred hatred of the God who had so fooled mankind. Life surged back into every artery and vein, full red blood, as there streamed out from me powerful and unchecked hatred and loathing for a master whose creation had been working wrongly for centuries and who was not wise enough, strong enough, or caring enough to mend it. I was livid with his apathy. Didn't he know what his carelessness had done to us? For the first time in my life I dared to demand an explanation.

When none came I was angrier than I ever remember being. I turned my eyes on the plain wooden cross and I remembered Calvary. I stood in the crowd that crucified him, hating and despising him. With my own hands I drove the nails into his hands and feet, and with bursting energy I flogged him and reviled him and spat with nauseating loathing. Now he should know what it felt like - to live in the creation he had made. Every breath brought from me the words: 'Now you know! Now you know!' And then I saw something which made my heart stand still. I saw his face, and on it twisted every familiar agony of my own soul. 'Now you know' became an awed whisper as I, motionless, watched his agony. 'Yes, now I know' was the passionate and pain-filled reply. 'Why else should I have come?' Stunned, I watched His eyes search desperately for the tiniest flicker of love in mine, and as we loved one another in the bleak and the cold, forsaken by God, frightened and derelict, we loved one another and our pain became silent in the calm.[4]

It is clear that when the woman poured out her anger against God, a repressed desire for God was not only released, it was satisfied by a new revelation of the Lord's presence in her painful vulnerability, and as a result the depression began to end. As William Blake once wrote, "I was angry with my friend, I told my wrath, my wrath did end. I was angry with my foe; I told it not, my wrath did grow."[5]

Conclusion

Besides helping clients to follow these steps, which would be familiar to counsellors and psycho-therapists, healers of course can pray, with the laying on of hands, for the relief of hurting memories which are so often the root cause of depression. As scripture assures us, "dear friends: With the Lord a day is like a thousand years, and a thousand years are like a day" (2 Pt 3:8). Even though those who suffered a trauma were not aware of the Lord's presence and help at the time the hurt or loss occurred, they can become aware of that comforting fact in a retrospective way, as they receive healing prayer in the present with expectant faith. It goes without saying, that healers can also pray for the relief of the other kinds of depression mentioned at the beginning of this chapter such as bipolar disorder and endogenous depression, while acknowledging that "nothing is impossible to God" (Lk 1:37). Those who suffer from any kind of depression can also have recourse to the sacrament of the anointing of the sick.

Before concluding this chapter it is worth mentioning that Christian spirituality talks about the inner experience of desolation

4   (London: Darton, Longman & Todd, 1982), 44.
5   "The Poison Tree" in *Songs of Innocence and of Experience*.

of spirit. Writing about it, in the fourth rule of his *Spiritual Exercises*, St Ignatius of Loyola described it's characteristics, "such as darkness of soul, disturbance in it, movement to low and earthly things, disquiet from various agitations and temptations, moving to lack of confidence, without hope, without love, finding oneself totally slothful, tepid, sad, and, as if separated from one's Creator and Lord." Although this sort of spiritual depression can be experienced at the same time as clinical depression, it is usually separate. A person could suffer from desolation of spirit without being clinically depressed. To be cured, desolation of spirit needs a spiritual remedy which could be recommended by a spiritual director, especially one who is familiar with Ignatian spirituality.[6]

6   Cf. Brigitte-Violaine Aufauvre, "Depression and Spiritual Desolation," *The Way*, 42/3 (July 2003), 47-56.

CHAPTER NINE

....

MINISTERING INNER HEALING

In a preceding chapter we looked at the need for inner healing for a lack of self-acceptance and low self-esteem which, as we noted, can have multiple causes and effects. In this chapter, we go on to suggest some ways, in which having experienced inner healing ourselves, we can minister that same type of healing to others, who will be referred to, in a slightly arbitrary way, in this chapter as the client/s. We can cooperate with the Spirit's healing work in three interrelated ways, namely, by encouraging the client to engage in honest self-disclosure to the healer and the Lord; by urging forgiveness of those who caused the victim's hurt by word, deed or omission; and by praying for healing of memories by means of the laying on of hands.[1]

Dispositions Needed

In order to be used by the Lord in inner healing, one has to ask for the grace to pray in the right spirit, i.e., a spirit of gentleness, compassion and reverence for the person. The one who prays for inner healing needs discernment in order to uncover what the root problem might be. To that end, one needs to ask God for the gift of wisdom mentioned in Is 11:2 and Jm 1:5-8. That prayer can be answered in a number of ways. Firstly, the healer may be enabled,

---

1   There are many good books on this subject such as, Barbara Shlemon, *Healing the Hidden Self* (Ann Arbor: Ave Maria Press, 2005); Matthew & Denis Linn, *Healing Life's Hurts: Healing Memories Through the Five Stages of Forgiveness* (New York: Paulist Press, 1977).

by means of perceptive, empathic questioning to go beyond a presenting problem, to discover what its root cause might be, e.g., a repressed, traumatic event in the past. Secondly, as a result of an intuitive hunch, which is often influenced by one's own past life experiences together with a knowledge of psychology, the healer might sense what the key issue really is. Thirdly, some healers are aided by a word of knowledge,[2] in the form of a mental picture or an inspired insight, e.g., of some forgotten or repressed memory. I can recall talking to a woman in her fifties and getting two accurate words of knowledge about her, the first was to do with the fact that she was suffering from an eating disorder and secondly, that it had been occasioned by her being sexually abused as a girl. It turned out that both words of knowledge were accurate. In this context it is worth noting that sometimes when a person asks for prayer for some physical problem, e.g., a diseased colon, the healer may sense that it is the presenting issue, whereas repressed anger, fear, guilt or shame to do with a past hurt is the real one. So the focus quickly switches from physical to inner healing.

Self-Disclosure and Inner Healing

Lack of self-acceptance leads to low self-esteem. If a client does suffer from a poor self-image, it is advisable to encourage him or her to talk about their problems. One urges them to tell the truth, the whole truth and nothing but the truth about their past memories and feelings, especially those which may be painful, shameful or embarrassing. As Jm 5:16 says, "confess your sins to one another, so that you may be healed." If a healer listens without any hint of judgement or condemnation and with "unconditional positive

---

2   It is a supernatural revelation of facts about a person or situation, which is not
     learned through the efforts of the natural mind, but is a fragment of knowl-
     edge freely given by God, disclosing the truth which the Spirit wishes to be
     made known concerning a particular person or situation.

regard,"[3] clients will begin to accept and love themselves as they are, and not as they have been pretending to be.[4]

For Catholics, one good way of doing this is to confess their wrongdoings in the sacrament of reconciliation. While Christians would not maintain that sickness and suffering are imposed by God on people as punishments for their personal sins, they would maintain that sickness and suffering can be a natural consequence of wrongdoing. Jesus implied as much when he healed the cripple at the pool of Bethesda, "See, you are well again. Stop sinning or something worse may happen to you" (Jn 5:14). St Paul made a similar point in 1 Cor 11:29-30 when he said, "those who eat and drink without discerning the body of Christ eat and drink judgment on themselves. That is why many among you are weak and sick." I think that Fr. Victor White, O.P., a friend of Carl Jung, was correct when he wrote, "while sacramental confession is not ordained to cure, it may do much to prevent, the disorders with which psychotherapy is concerned."[5] For example, lay friends of mine have told me that sometimes when they meet fellow Catholics who are suffering from all kinds of mental health problems, they encourage them to make a good general confession to a priest. They have also told me that, in some instances, when their advice was followed, some people have reported being inwardly transformed, presumably because a weight of corrosive moral guilt has been lifted from their hearts and replaced by a reassuring sense of God's presence and peace.

At graced moments of self-disclosure like the ones described, one could imagine that the fiery dove of the Spirit alights in people's hearts in an affirming manner, as the Giver of Life who releases

---

3   A phrase associated with Carl Rogers a pioneer of counselling theory. It refers to the basic acceptance and support of a person regardless of what the person says or does, especially in the context of client-centred therapy.

4   This is the thinking that informs step five of AA, "We admitted to God, to ourselves, *and to another human being* the exact nature of our wrongs."

5   *God and the Unconscious* (Glasgow: Fontana, 1952), 186.

inner strength, healing and tranquillity. To paraphrase Eph 2:14-17, at moments like that the dividing wall of rejection breaks down between the acceptable and the unacceptable self in a liberating way. As a result of getting back in touch with the innermost self, new energy of a positive kind is made available to the personality and a Christian sense of self-esteem is nurtured.

If clients have suffered some kind of trauma/s, healers can assist the victims, as best they can, to remember the hurtful experiences and their associated feelings which are often repressed, rationalized, or projected outward in the form of dysfunctional attitudes and behaviours. Frequently, as we have already noted, those negative feelings will be pushed down into the unconscious. For instance, some men and women have been brought up to feel that all anger is sinful, e.g., because Jesus said, "I tell you that anyone who is angry with a brother or sister will be subject to judgment" (Mt 5:22).[6] Consequently they are afraid to express their anger, as we saw in chapter eight on overcoming depression. Repressed feelings of antagonism and resentment don't go away. They are simply buried alive in the unconscious where they attack the person while suppressing his or her sense of conscious relationship with the Lord. It can also be noted, in passing, that un-forgiveness can give evil spirits a foothold which will be exploited at the hurt person's expense. So the healer, encourages the client, with God's help, to try to recall hurting memories, to recover their associated feelings, while going on to express them openly and honestly, firstly in a private journal, secondly to the healer in dialogue and thirdly, to God in prayer. As a proverb says, "a problem shared is a problem halved."

Forgiveness and Inner Healing

Lack of forgiveness and resentment against the people, living or dead, who hurt a client, and against an apparently uncaring God who allowed the hurt to happen, is another common problem. In

6   The feeling of anger is not sinful in itself. It is what we do to express anger that may be sinful. Scripture says, "Be angry, and do not sin" (Eph 4:26).

psychological and spiritual terms there is only one way forward, and that is by means of forgiveness. While it is true that divine forgiveness is freely available to sinners at all times, a client can only truly experience that forgiveness to the extent that he or she is willing to forgive those who have hurt or injured them. The scriptures make this abundantly clear. We can take a brief look at a representative text. In Lk 6:36-39 Jesus says, "Do not judge and you will not be judged; do not condemn and you will not be condemned. Forgive and you will be forgiven ... for the measure you give will be the measure you will get back." If there is someone who a client needs to forgive he or she could react in three possible ways "I won't," "I can't," or "I will with God's help."

Willingness to forgive the living and the dead is God's way forward into Christian healing, wholeness and peace. Healers can assure their clients that when such a willingness is present, it is not only in conformity with the will of God, the Holy Spirit will be poured out upon them, thereby enabling them to cross the bridge from resentment to forgiveness. When the time seems right, the healer can lead the client in saying something like this prayer. By the way, in the past I have sometimes knelt down and urged the client to do the same while saying together,

"Father in heaven, in the name of Jesus your divine and merciful Son, help me to worship you in spirit and in truth. Take away my heart of stone and grant me, instead, a merciful heart like yours. Forgive me for the many times I have hurt you and other people. Help me, in my turn, to be merciful as you are merciful by forgiving this person/s who stands in need of my forgiveness. And now Lord having given me the desire to forgive (*mention the name/s*) from my heart, grant me the power to do so by your Holy Spirit. I thank you that even now you are granting me the grace of forgiveness, taking away my bitterness, and releasing and blessing the person who hurt me in the past. Amen"

It is admirable when people who have suffered a terrible loss declare afterwards how they have forgiven those who were responsible. That said, healers need to warn their clients that if a hurt goes deep, it will normally be associated with many negative feelings which need to be fully acknowledged over a period of time. If they are suppressed in the name of a premature and dutiful act of forgiveness, there is a danger that the subsequent forgiveness will be superficial and lacking depth and effectiveness. As the onion of pain is progressively peeled, with the aid of a healer and introspection, new layers of hurt and anger will be exposed, hence the scriptural injunction that victims need to keep on forgiving, (cf. Mt 18:22) until no anger or resentment remains.[7]

Prayer for Healing of Hurting Memories

People who unconsciously espouse the just world hypothesis, assume that a person's good actions will be rewarded by good fortune. However, they can feel betrayed when God allows them to experience misfortune instead. Understandably, they ask the question, like Job of old, "I live a good life, why did God not prevent this happening to me, why didn't he care for me? I thought he not only looks after the birds of the air, but that he promises to look after his children in a special way" (cf. Mt 6:26). When people have hurting memories, these are very understandable questions. At this point the healer should encourage the disillusioned client to honestly express his or her negative feelings of anger and even rage to God. Then a number of truths need to be clarified in order to proceed.

Firstly, people were created with freedom. As a result, God does not interfere with that freedom even if it is used in a hurtful or harmful way. Secondly, God loves all of us, and when we were being hurt or harmed, the loving heart of God was, and is, grieved to see us suffer. As Gen 6:6 says, "The Lord was grieved... and his

---

7   For an extended forgiveness prayer see Appendix five below.

heart was filled with pain." Thirdly, it says in scripture that as far as God is concerned our sense of chronological time, is an eternal, timeless now. It means that when a Christian prays for the healing of hurting memories, he or she invites the Lord to revisit those hurting memories while saying to a client, "while you were not aware of God's love when these bad things happened to you, that love was there at the time. It will touch your memories right now and reveal the compassionate love the Lord had and still has for you. The experience of that love will help to heal your painful memories and bring you peace." Strange as it may seem clients can be urged to thank God, not for the hurt/s themselves, but in the belief that they were not only embraced by the providence of God, God will not allow evil to have the last word. It belongs to God and it will be a word of blessing. As St Paul says, "give thanks in *all* circumstances; for this is God's will for you in Christ Jesus" (1 Thess 5:18).[8]

Afterwards the healer goes on to pray, usually accompanied by the gentle laying on of hands,[9] about specific memories which the person has revealed, together with their associated negative feelings. As St Paul said in Eph 3:16, "I ask God from the wealth of his glory to give you power through his Spirit to be strong in your inner selves." This kind of prayer takes time. In this regard, the following two points are helpful. Firstly, while one focuses on the client's experience, one also listens to the Lord while seeking divine guidance. Secondly, when a healer doesn't quite know specifically what to pray for, he or she can resort to praying in tongues. As St Paul said, "we do not know what to pray for as we ought, but the Spirit himself intercedes for us with groans too deep for words. And he who searches hearts knows what is the mind of the Spirit, because the Spirit intercedes for the saints according to the will of God" (Rm 8:26-27). I have found that there is real power in

---

8   For more on this subject see chapter eight.
9   Not everyone is comfortable being touched, so it is important to ask the client's permission to do so.

this kind of prayer and that it is sometimes accompanied by spontaneous inspirations of a helpful kind such as a relevant scripture text, and sometimes a word of knowledge. Occasionally, a client will need to be prayed with for inner healing on a number of occasions. This is referred to as soaking prayer.

Conclusion

During the many years of my priestly ministry I have found that in Western countries the main manner in which people experience poverty of spirit is in psycho-spiritual ways. That poverty, when acknowledged is a vulnerable place where God can be encountered by means of inner healing. As Jesus promised, "Blessed are the poor in Spirit" (Mt 5:3), i.e., happy those who because of their awareness of vulnerability, need and hurt open their hearts to God's healing self-communication in the Holy Spirit. It is the privilege of those who minister inner healing, to evangelise in this compassionate way. I have found on a number of occasions that when I and others have prayed for inner healing, the man or woman also experienced a psychosomatic healing, e.g., I can remember a man's leg being healed in Derry when he forgave a driver who had caused his disability; and I can also recall a woman getting relief from arthritic pain when she was prayed with for healing of an unresolved grief to do with her mother's death many years before.

....

Chapter Ten

The Father Wound

Speaking about the role of fathers in family life, Dr. David Popenoe, a sociologist in Rutgers University in the USA, said in his book *Life Without the Father*, "Fathers are far more than just "second adults" in the home. Involved fathers – especially biological ones – bring positive benefits to their children that no other person is as likely to bring. They provide protection and economic support and male role models. They have a parenting style that is significantly different from that of a mother and that difference is important in healthy child development . . . Fathers encourage competition, engendering independence. Mothers promote equity, creating a sense of security. Dads emphasize conceptual communication, which helps kids expand their vocabulary and intellectual capacities. Moms major in sympathy, care, and help, thus demonstrating the importance of relationships. Dads tend to see their child in relation to the rest of the world. Moms tend to see the rest of the world in relation to their child."[1]

With this in mind, we can note how on February 16th, 2008, Cardinal Carlo Caffara of Bologna reported that he had received a relatively long letter from Sr Lucia of Fatima in which she said prophetically, "the final battle between the Lord and the reign of Satan will be about marriage and the family." Speaking to Charismatics gathered in Rome's Olympic Stadium in 2014, Pope Francis echoed that sentiment when he said, "Families are the domestic church where Jesus grows in the love of a married couple, in the lives of their children. This is why the devil attacks the family so much. The devil doesn't

---

1   (New York: The Free Press, 1996), 163.

want it and tries to destroy it. The devil tries to make love disappear from the family." One of the widespread problems faced by families, at present, is the phenomenon of the absent father. Pope Francis spoke about this state of affairs in his Apostolic Exhortation *The Joy of Love*. In Par. 55 he wrote, "The absence of a father gravely affects family life and the upbringing of children and their integration into society. This absence, which may be physical, emotional, psychological and spiritual, deprives children of a suitable father figure."

Physical Absence

Let's begin by looking at the phenomenon of physically absent fathers. It can take many forms. Firstly, there seems to be an ever-increasing number of unmarried mothers. Once the father has participated in the conception of a child he moves away and leaves the rearing of the baby to the mother. Secondly, sad to say, there are fathers, who die when their child or children are still quite young. A nun in England told me how her father died in one room on the very day that she was born in another. Thirdly, there are an increasing number of fathers who are separated or divorced and who live away from their children. Fourthly, there are fathers who have to live away from home for long periods of time, e.g., because of being in prison, or serving overseas in the armed forces, working in another country, or being part of a ship's crew, etc. Fifthly, nowadays lesbian couples raise children. From a psychological and emotional point of view, the kids will be at a disadvantage due to the absence of a father. There are other fathers who in spite of the fact that they live at home are rarely there because of the length of time they spend in their workplace and the periods they devote to other activities outside the home, such as sport. One American website makes the disturbing observation that before they reach the age of eighteen, more than half of all children are likely to spend at least a significant portion of their childhoods living apart from their fathers.[2]

---

2   https://thefathercode.com/the-9-devastating-effects-of-the-absent-father/

Emotional Absence

There are other fathers who, although they are physically present, are emotionally absent. Many dads lack emotional self-awareness and as a result find it hard to express their feelings even when they are aware of them. They may also suffer from such inhibiting things as depression, anxiety states, ill-health, addictions and the like. As a result, they don't talk much to their children in a personal way. They don't embrace them or tell them they love them. They are usually slow to affirm or praise them. Some fathers are authoritarian, controlling and hard to please. Others in spite of being good providers are distant, non-demonstrative, and fairly uncommunicative about their past lives. When their children want to confide in a parent, they usually talk to their mother rather than their father.

Sad to say there are fathers, who are not only emotionally detached, they may be abusive, *physically* by using violence on their wives and/or children, e.g., when they have been drinking; *emotionally*, by means of put-downs, criticism, invidious comparisons, disparaging remarks, e.g., "you are stupid and a born loser;" and *sexually*, by means of inappropriate activity of one kind or another, e.g., carelessly leaving porn DVDs within reach of children; and *spiritually*, by making negative comments about religious faith and practices or by talking about God in scary terms as someone who is hard to please, harsh and vindictive.

Here are ten predictable effects of the Father wound whether due to physical and emotional absence, or abuse of one kind or another.

1) Their children will be five times more likely, than the average, to commit suicide.
2) They will be subject to dramatically increased rates of depression and anxiety.
3) They will be liable to decreased education achievement and increased drop-out rates.
4) Consistently lower average income levels.
5) Lower job security.
6) Increased rates of divorce and relationship issues.

7) Substantially increased rates of substance abuse.
8) Increases in social and mental behavioural issues.
9) Twice as likely to suffer from obesity.
10) More likely to commit crime and to go to prison.

Apropos of the last point, there is an account of how a famous card company provided free Mother's Day cards to U.S. prison inmates so they could send one to their mums. Almost every prisoner lined up eagerly to receive a card. The event was so successful, the company decided to do the same thing for Father's Day. But the results were quite different. No one wanted a card. It seems that either the inmates didn't have a father or their father was not someone they wanted to contact.

Some effects of the father wound on daughters

Daughters need their fathers to love, cherish and affirm them as persons and as females. But if the father-daughter relationship does not have a chance to fully develop then the young girl may adopt negative beliefs about herself and develop unrealistic perceptions and expectations to do with the men in her life. Psychotherapists have noted four effects of an absent father on their daughters. Firstly, girls who grew up with an emotionally absent father often develop an anxious attachment style, causing them to feel preoccupied with their romantic relationships. Secondly, women who behave this way are subconsciously living in a state of fear and distrust. They struggle with the fear of being abandoned and are at a higher risk of dissatisfaction in relationships because they would rather be in a dysfunctional relationship than to be alone. It's common for these women to end up in abusive partnerships and to accept abusive behaviour. Thirdly, if a girl doesn't get enough attention or doesn't feel really valued, especially in her relationship with her dad, she will grow up and seek that attention from other men. Eventually a clinging neediness will push the woman's partner away, which in turn will confirm her greatest fear—that she is unlovable and unwanted. Fourthly, trust is a *major* component of positive emotional attachment. When a girl hasn't experienced the love, affection, and protection of a loving man, as a woman she is more likely to develop defences or protective mechanisms that will keep her separated from them in some way. As an adult, she may crave closeness and intimacy but then she will be inclined to push it away to protect herself from possible hurt and rejection.[3]

Some effects of the father wound on sons

As far as sons are concerned, they need their father's love, affirmation and encouragement too, not only to develop healthy self-esteem but also to grow in a confident way into their male identity, role and responsibilities. But if they suffer from the father wound, due to an absent or inadequate father, then they are more likely to lack such things as a sense of worthiness throughout their lives. The son acquires a profound distrust of the continuity and stability of relationships. Abandoned men habitually have relationship difficulties with their parents, siblings, chosen partners, and their own children. Sons who had an absent father are more likely to leave their own families and thus perpetuate the vicious cycle of abandonment. Sons without a father are also more likely to divorce as adults and also more likely to be unfaithful. Boys and men with an orphan spirit are more likely to suffer from anger, anxiety, loneliness and passivity. They will also have an unconscious propensity to develop unhealthy attitudes and behaviours, such as drinking too much, taking drugs, gambling, having recourse to pornography and a negative attitude to people in authority etc.

Conclusion

When children have a physically absent father, I've found that a good man, such as a grandfather, uncle, family friend or step father can act as a father substitute, someone who lovingly mentors the

---

3   Cf. https://verilymag.com/2017/08/daddy-issues-how-our-fathers-
     impact-our-relationships

children of a family in a consistent, and committed way. By doing so, the father substitute can mitigate any harm that might otherwise have been done by the absence of the children's biological father. Psychological studies have indicated that good father figures can have a significantly positive role in the development of children. Other men, such as teachers, sports coaches, clergymen, and neighbours can act as good role models, especially for boys, by role modelling how to be a good man, father or husband.

CHAPTER ELEVEN

....

THE FATHER WOUND AND FALSE IMAGES OF GOD

In his excellent book *The Central Message of the New Testament*, eminent Lutheran scholar Joachim Jermias devoted the first section to a discussion of the unique importance of Jesus' use of Abba as a form of address to God, his Father.[1] Jeremias returned to the same subject in his *New Testament Theology*. He stated there that, "The use of the everyday word 'abba' as a form of address to God is the most important linguistic innovation on the part of Jesus."[2] Apparently, the word 'abba' does not mean "dear father," "papa" or "dadda" The more accurate translation would be "the father," or "my father." Later Jeremias added, "The complete novelty and uniqueness of 'Abba' as an address to God in the prayer of Jesus shows that it expresses the heart of Jesus' relationship to God. He spoke to God as a child to its father: confidently and securely, and yet at the same time reverently and obediently."[3] Jeremias went on to add that this form of address was not confined to small children, grown-up sons and daughters also addressed their fathers as 'abba.'

Pope Francis said in par. 176 of his Apostolic Exhortation, *The Joy of Love*, "We often hear that ours is 'a society without fathers.' In Western culture, the father figure is said to be symbolically absent, missing or vanished. Manhood itself seems to be called into

1   (London: SCM, 1965), 8-30.
2   (London: SCM, 1981),, 36.
3   Ibid., 67.

question. The result has been an understandable confusion. At first, this was perceived as a liberation: liberation from the father as master, from the father as the representative of a law imposed from without, from the father as the arbiter of his children's happiness and an obstacle to the emancipation and autonomy of young people. In some homes authoritarianism once reigned and, at times, even oppression."[4]

Effects of the father wound on relationship with God

Apart from the well-documented psychological and sociological disadvantages associated with the crisis of fatherhood, there can be religious consequences also. We get to know something about the Fatherhood of God from our human fathers. As Pope John Paul II said in *Man and Woman He Created Them: A Theology of the Body*, "The body, in fact, and only the body, is capable of making visible what is invisible: the spiritual and the divine. It has been created to transfer into the visible reality of the world the mystery hidden from eternity in God, and thus to be a sign of it."[5] All adults can reflect what God the Father is like, especially biological fathers. The extent to which right relationship with one's father is lacking is the extent to which God's presence can be distorted or eclipsed.

Pope Benedict adverted to this problem when he said in January 2013, "It is not always easy today to talk about fatherhood. Especially in our Western world, broken families, increasingly absorbing work commitments, concerns, and often the fatigue of trying to balance the family budget, and the distracting invasion of the mass media in daily life are some of the many factors that can prevent a peaceful and constructive relationship between fathers and their children. At times communication becomes difficult, trust can be lost and relationships with the father figure can become problematic. Even imagining God as a father becomes difficult, not having had adequate models of reference. For those who have had the experience

4   Catechesis (28 January 2015) in *L'Osservatore Romano*, 29 Jan 2015, 8.
5   (Boston: Pauline Books & Media, 2006), 203.

of an overly authoritarian and inflexible father, or an indifferent father lacking in affection, or even an absent father, it is not easy to think of God as Father and trustingly surrender oneself to Him."[6]

The views of psychologists

Psychologists, such as Dr Ana-Maria Rizzuto a Catholic psychoanalyst from Argentina, say that most people have *ideas* and *images* of God.[7] We get our ideas from the instruction given by our parents, teachers, priests etc. They are usually positive. They say that God is great, all powerful, loving, forgiving, etc. Our images of God are based on our childhood experience of parental authority, and caring. If a child's father was absent or abusive, in the ways we have already mentioned, the child will tend to form negative images of God. Spiritual directors are familiar with the fact that our images of God can have a significant but unconscious influence on our relationship with God the Father and our way of praying.

Dr Rizzuto has described how a parish priest came to see her. His presenting symptoms were chronic fatigue and insomnia which lessened his ability to be available to his parishioners. A thorough examination revealed that there was nothing wrong with him physically. However, when Rizzuto asked the priest about his family it became clear from his tone of voice that, although he admired his father, he also feared him because he was sometimes stern, demanding and punitive. When she asked the priest about his relationship with God his reply was ambiguous. As Rizzuto observed, the God of the priest's professed theology was loving, patient and gentle. However, the God of the man's operative theology was critical, stern and demanding. Dr. Rizzuto went on to describe how she helped the priest to consciously recognize the conflict between his *idea* and his *image* of God, and how the former was the fruit of his education and the latter a result of his childhood experience of

6   General Audience, Reflections on the Creed.
7   Cf. Ana-Maria Rizzuto, *Birth of the Living God: A Psychoanalytic Study* (Chicago: Chicago University Press, 1981).

paternal authority. As soon as he became aware of these conflicting aspects of his relationship with God, the priest was able, over a period of time, to revise his image of the Lord and to overcome his feeling of resistance.

American psychologist, Paul Vitz, has shown in his book, *Faith of the Fatherless: The Psychology of Atheism*,[8] how many prominent and influential non-believers such as Nietzsche, Hume, Russell, Freud, Sartre, Camus and Feuerbach, had a dysfunctional relationship with their earthly fathers. As a result of what he calls the defective father hypothesis, they could not affirm the fact that the heavenly Father exists. Vitz said in the course of an interview, "Fathers are very important in the religious life of their children; in particular, good fathers are a major contributor to the probability that their children will be believers and that bad fathers or dysfunctional fathers have the opposite effect. Being a dysfunctional father, that is, not being present, not being supportive, or being abusive; all of these things tend to make children back away from the notion of God as father on a psychological level and thus never get through to religious belief in God."[9]

No Longer Orphans

In his book, *Sonship: A Journey into Father's Heart* New Zealand author James Jordan includes a very interesting reflection on some words of Jesus in Jn 14:18, "I will not leave you orphans, I will come to you." He interprets what Jesus promised in a novel way.[10] Firstly, he suggests that when Satan and other angels rebelled, in effect they were saying, "We do not want a father over us, we want to be the father. No one is going to be over us. We are not sons or daughters, we are not subject to anybody." In other words, Satan and the fallen angels are orphans and want us to be spiritual orphans also. Secondly, when Satan successfully tempted Adam and Eve, and through them

8   (San Francisco: Ignatius Press, 2013).
9   http://www.fathersforgood.org/ffg/en/big_four/faith_fatherless.html
10   (Taupo, New Zealand: Tree of Life Media, 2012), 115-140.

the whole human race, "In leaving the garden," as Jordan says, "they were leaving the environment of the Father's love and becoming more like the one cast out of heaven. They were becoming fatherless... In them the whole human race was becoming orphaned."[11] We sinners have all shared in that orphan spirit. It is our primordial problem. But Jesus promised, "I will not leave you orphans."

God the Father is the prototype of all fatherhood, not our human fathers, who merely mirror or fail to mirror what God is like. As St Paul says in Eph 3:14, "I kneel before the Father from whom every family in heaven and on earth derives its name." That being so, St Paul prayed in Eph 1:17, "I keep asking that the God of our Lord Jesus Christ, the glorious Father, may give you the Spirit of wisdom and revelation, *so that you may know him better*." That prayer is answered when people are enabled to develop a loving personal relationship with Jesus, principally, by means of being baptised in the Holy Spirit and praying the scriptures in a contemplative way. As Jn 1:14 says, "The Word became a human being and, full of grace and truth, lived among us. We saw his glory, the glory which he received as the Father's only Son." It was he who said that he is our Way to the Father (cf. Jn 14:6). In this manner, people who suffer from the orphan spirit and the related father wound can be helped to progressively replace their negative images of God the Father with more realistic, positive ones. This is a work of the Spirit who leads us to pray "Abba, dear Father."

The Father's Love Letter

My Child, you may not know me, but I know everything about you (Ps 139:1). I know when you sit down and when you rise up (Ps 139:2). I am familiar with all your ways (Ps 139:3)—even the very hairs on your head are numbered (Matt 10:29–31).

You were made in my image (Gen 1:27). In me you live and move and have your being, for you are my offspring (Acts 17:28). I

---

11   Ibid., 139.

knew you even before you were conceived (Jer 1:4–5). I chose you when I planned creation (Eph 1:11–12). You were not a mistake, for all your days are written in my book (Ps 139:15–16). I determined the exact time of your birth and where you would live (Acts 17:26). You are fearfully and wonderfully made (Ps 139:14). I knit you together in your mother's womb (Ps 139:13), and brought you forth on the day you were born (Ps 71:6).

I have been misrepresented by those who don't know me (John 8:41–44). I am not distant and angry, but am the complete expression of love (1 John 4:16). And it is my desire to lavish my love on you (1 John 3:1), simply because you are my child and I am your Father (1 John 3:1). I offer you more than your earthly father ever could (Matt 7:11), for I am the perfect Father (Matt 5:48). Every good gift that you receive comes from my hand (James 1:17), for I am your provider and I meet all your needs (Matt 6:31–33).

My plan for your future has always been filled with hope (Jer 29:11), because I love you with an everlasting love (Jer 31:3). My thoughts toward you are as countless as the sand on the seashore (Ps 139:17–18), and I rejoice over you with singing (Zeph 3:17). I will never stop doing good to you (Jer 32:40), for you are my treasured possession (Ex 19:5).

I desire to establish you with all my heart and all my soul (Jer 32:41), and I want to show you great and marvellous things (Jer 33:3). If you seek me with all your heart, you will find me (Deut 4:29); delight in me and I will give you the desires of your heart (Ps 37:4), for it is I who gave you those desires (Phil 2:13).

I am able to do more for you than you could possibly imagine (Eph 3:20), for I am your greatest encourager (2 Thess 2:16–17). I am also the Father who comforts you in all your troubles (2 Cor 1:3–4). When you are broken hearted, I am close to you (Ps 34:18); as a shepherd carries a lamb, I have carried you close to my heart (Isa 40:11). One day I will wipe away every tear from your eyes, and I will take away all the pain you have suffered on this earth (Rev 21:3–4).

I am your Father, and I love you even as I love my son, Jesus (John 17:23). In him, my love for you is revealed (John 17:26). He is the exact representation of my being (Heb 1:3). He came to demonstrate that I am for you, not against you (Rom 8:31), and to tell you that I am not counting your sins against you (2 Cor 5:18–19). Jesus died so that you and I could be reconciled (2 Cor 5:18–19). His death was the ultimate expression of my love for you (1 John 4:10): I gave up everything I loved that I might gain your love (Rom 8:31–32).

If you receive the gift of my son, Jesus, you receive me (1 John 2:23), and nothing will ever separate you from my love again (Rom 8:38–39). Come home and I'll throw the biggest party heaven has ever seen (Luke 15:7). I have always been Father and will always be Father (Eph 3:14–15). My question is: will you be my child (John 1:12–13)? I am waiting for you (Luke 15:11–32).122

Love, Your Dad (Almighty God)

12 https://www.fathersloveletter.com/
For a recording https://www.fathersloveletter.com/audio.html

CHAPTER TWELVE

THE MOTHER WOUND

The Barnardo's Homes have a saying which states that, 'Every childhood lasts a lifetime.' A psychologist like Frank Lake argued that this is not only true, the story begins in the womb. In his book, *With Respect: A Doctor's Response to a Healing Pope*, he wrote, "What happens in the womb is of the utmost importance to the mental health and personality structure of the next generation. The emotional state of both parents is crucial, since the father's mood and passion carries across to his wife. What immediately affects and is imprinted upon the foetus are the flux of the mother's emotions."[1] He went on to suggest that, "where resentful emotions are aroused and violent actions undertaken which invite retribution, this creates the worst possible environment for the rooting of the next generation."[2]

Freud believed that once a child is born all the basic emotional attitudes which will influence it for a lifetime are in place by the age of six. Psychologists say that very early in it's life a child experiences symbiotic union with the mother, i.e., a merging of identities so that the pronouns "I" and "you" are not really differentiated. While being breast fed satisfies his or her biological needs, the child is being fed emotionally and spiritually, mainly by the quality of the mother's love and what psychologists refer to as attunement. The mother may speak, the baby may gurgle, but basically there is not an exchange

1   (London: Darton, Longman & Todd, 1986), 120. On page xix he wrote, "There is widespread medical support for the new awareness that maternal emotional disturbance distresses the foetus, leading to ill-effects that are detectable postnatally and on into adult life. It comes from embryologists, foetologists, obstetricians, paediatricians and epidemiologists, and from other independent workers."

2   Ibid., 120.

of thoughts. Rather the child is enwombed psychologically, and its identity is established in the reflected light of the mother's love. The extent to which that sense of love is defective and conditional is the extent to which the child's sense of self-acceptance and self-esteem will be compromised and weakened. Neurotics, as was noted in chapter seven, have only conditional love for themselves. There are many possible causes for this. We will mention a few of them which are related to the quality of relationship with the mother.

Childhood separation

Sometimes a child gets the impression that it is not really very lovable, because of being separated from its parents, especially the mother. There can be many reasons for this. Firstly, the child may be born prematurely. As a result, it is kept in a hospital incubator and so deprived of physical contact and bonding with its mother. Or it may be that the child may have to go to hospital in its first few years. The mother visits, then she goes away again. The child can feel rejected. If it does, it blames itself. It feels, "There must be something wrong with me, that is why my mother keeps on leaving me!" Secondly, it may be that the mother herself has to go to hospital for an extended period. She might even die. The child doesn't understand this. It feels deserted and abandoned. As a result it suffers from what psychologists call separation anxiety, a feeling that can keep on resurfacing in adult life. Thirdly, sometimes a sick or pregnant mother will send one of her children to stay with a grandmother or aunt for a year or two, or even permanently. In some of those cases the child may get the mistaken impression that it was given away, because it wasn't wanted. This impression can have a detrimental effect on self-esteem.

Conditional love

A child is a bundle of selfish needs and desires. Naturally the parents try to fit it into the life of the family and to prevent it causing damage or disruption. Sometimes in the course of disciplining the child, a mother can give the impression that her love is conditional. It depends on the child's willingness to do as he or she is told. The mother's words, tone of voice and facial features can say to the child, "I'll love you more if... if you do as I say, if you don't go into temper tantrums" etc. In the child's mind this can give the impression that, "I'm lovable for what I do, and not for who I am." We know that as children get older, they internalise these attitudes. Consequently, they end up by only being able to love and accept themselves when they do their duty, what they "ought, should, must do." If they do something contrary to their moral code, they withdraw approval and love from themselves, thereby evoking separation anxiety and possibly unhealthy, morbid guilt of a neurotic, scrupulous kind.

Lack of Affirmation

Many parents and teachers can be too critical of their children. They are inclined to find fault and to expect the worst, while neglecting to show appreciation, and confident expectation. I can remember asking my mother what her initial impression was when she saw me for the first time. She was reluctant to respond. She said, "you might not like my answer." "Tell me anyway," I replied. "Well," she said, "when the nurse put you in my arms I thought to myself, his mouth is too big." It was typical of her attitude. She would continue as she began. All through my life I was used to her saying, "That was good ... but...and then would follow a criticism." No doubt she loved me, but she was a perfectionist, and as such was acutely aware of my faults and failings. Instead of seeing my life as if it were a sheet of white paper with a blob on it, she saw a blue blob on white paper. She justified her reluctance to offer praise because she would say, "It leads people to have swelled heads, and pride, the greatest of sins, precedes a fall." As a result, of maternal attitudes like these, self-esteem is damaged and the child fails to develop his or her potential. The same kind of thing can find an amplifying echo in adult life. A person's best efforts are taken for granted, but as soon as he or she makes a mistake they hear all about it from other people. The effect is not only discouraging; it can also reinforce a bad self-image.

Narcissistic Personality

Some mothers, suffer from narcissistic personality disorder, a problem characterised by a need for admiration while suffering from a lack of empathy for others. A person with this condition may have a grandiose sense of self-importance, a sense of entitlement, and take advantage of others. Speaking about his narcissistic mother, well-known psychologist Abraham Maslow wrote these shocking words, "What I reacted against and totally hated and rejected was not only her physical appearance, but also her values and world view, her stinginess, her total selfishness, her lack of love for anyone else in the world, even her own husband and children, her narcissism, her anti-Negro prejudice, her exploitation of anyone, her assumption that anyone was wrong who disagreed with her, her lack of concern for her grandchildren, her lack of friends, her sloppiness and dirtiness, her lack of family feeling for her own parents and siblings, her primitive animal-like care for herself and her body alone etc, etc."[3] The experience of being raised by a narcissistic mother leads to low self-esteem, inability to form healthy relationships, a need for perfection, and lapses into extreme self-criticism. This, in turn, leads to a hollow sense of self, known as a *"false self."* These children are drained of their energy and often dismissed and/or punished when they don't fulfil their mother's needs and wishes.

Lack of affection

For one reason or another, a mother may be unable to give a child the love it needs. If she is suffering from an emotional problem, e.g., post natal depression, mental illness or addiction she will tend to be self-absorbed and won't have the ability to give the child enough affection. Sometimes a mother's energies are absorbed with the

3   Edward Hoffman, *The Right to be Human* (Wellingborough: Crucible, 1989), 9.

difficult task of coping with a troublesome husband. Worry about such things as paying bills, mental health problems and possible violence from her partner can create an atmosphere of tension and fear. This kind of environment generates anxiety and insecurity, not self-esteem in the children. Single mothers can lack quality time with their children because of having to work long hours in order to earn enough money to finance the home. Lastly, some mothers have more children than they can really care for. As a result, one or more of them may feel neglected from an emotional point of view. Even in smaller families, children can feel much the same, because their mothers are unable to express physical affection to them or to say the words, "I love you."

Some signs of the mother wound

Adults dealing with a mother wound often look back on their child-hood and can identify issues such as:

- Never feeling they had their mother's approval or acceptance.
- Concerns about not being loved by their mother or not being loved as much as other siblings or family members.
- Difficulties in relating to the mother on an emotional level.
- Uncertainty about the relationship with the mother and if it could be lost with a mistake or an accident.
- Always trying to do better or to be perfect, in order to attempt to gain your mother's attention and acceptance.
- Feelings of having to protect, care for, or shelter your mother rather than her protecting, caring for and sheltering you.

Conclusion

The purpose of this chapter was not to judge or condemn mothers for their shortcomings. In my experience their failings, more often than not, are due to weakness rather than malice. The majority of mothers, not only love their children as best they can with their limited inner resources, they express that love within the confines of their modest abilities. Children who come to acknowledge that they are suffering from the mother wound are urged, in their adult years, to recall what their experience of being mothered was like, not in order to criticise, but rather to understand. It is done as a prelude to receiving the sort of healing which would facilitate their growth into a greater capacity to love in a self-forgetful, empathic way.

Due to the limitations of space, I have said very little about the different ways in which the mother wound effects sons and daughters. Put briefly it can be said that daughters who suffer from this wound often lack confidence; form unhealthy attachments in relationships; suffer from hyper sensitivity, as well as lacking trust and a sense of boundaries. Sons who suffer from the mother wound can be ambivalent toward women. On the one hand they need them, but on the other they are wary of them. They can remain emotionally fused to their mothers in an unhealthy way, or else become detached in a stance of defensive protection. When their wives disappoint them, they can feel profound letdown and even rage.

A common objection to facing the painful implications of the mother wound is, "we should let sleeping dogs lie." However, we can never truly escape from, or bury the past. It lives on in the present, albeit at an unconscious level. If we avoid dealing with the pain associated with one of the most primary and foundational relationships in our lives, it will inevitably subvert and distort our current relationships thereby causing us to miss an important opportunity to discover the truth of who we really are and to authentically and joyfully realise our potential.

CHAPTER THIRTEEN

....

HEALING THE FATHER & MOTHER WOUND

Because we love our parents many of us tend to idealise them by putting them on an unrealistic pedestal of perfection. As a result we tend to either overlook or excuse their shortcomings and weaknesses. We need to be realistic about the ways in which, despite their best intentions, they may have failed to meet our legitimate needs. It is important to acknowledge one's consequential feelings of loss, pain, anger etc. The aim here, as was said before, is to understand rather than to blame, judge or condemn.

Shakespeare wrote, "since you know you cannot see yourself so well as by reflection, I, your glass, will modestly discover to yourself, that of yourself which you yet know not of."[1] Given that those words are true, it can be helpful to speak to a trusted friend, a trained counsellor, therapist or spiritual director. They can help you to get in touch with your unknown self, i.e., the repressed and unacknowledged aspects of the father or mother wound, and its consequences, in a context of confidentiality and loving psychological safety. In order to experience healing of the parental wound a number of things can be done.

Praise and thanksgiving

Firstly, while acknowledging our negative memories and feelings we try to go beyond a purely victim mentality by means of praise and thanksgiving for everything, even one's misfortunes (cf. 1 Thess 5:17-18; Eph 5:20). Having acknowledged our negative feelings,

....

1   *Julius Caesar*, Act 1, scene 2, line 70.

we should thank God for the graces and blessings of life and like Paul and Silas in prison, start praising God instead of wallowing in pain, resentment or anger. St Paul implied that we should thank God for the bad things. How can we thank the Lord for the sins and misfortunes in our lives? It is not that we thank God *for* these evils in themselves, but because we believe that they have been embraced by God's loving providence. God can bring good from evil, as God did from Christ's crucifixion. What began as a painful inner state will be transformed by the milk of God's mercy and love, into a beautiful pearl of great price.[2]

Anthony de Mello, S.J., said in his book *Sadhana: A Way to God* that if he were to choose the one form of prayer that made Christ's healing presence most real in his life it would be the prayer of thanksgiving. He explained, "The prayer consists, quite simply in thanking God for everything. It is based on the belief that nothing happens in our life that is not foreseen and planned by God – just nothing, not even our sins."[3] As St Paul testified, "Where sin abounds, grace abounds much more." (Rm 5:20).

Merlin Carothers, a Methodist minister, wrote a number of influential books about praising and thanking God in all circumstances.[4] His thesis was simple, biblical and powerful. Firstly, he said quite rightly that, God has a perfect plan for our lives, but cannot move us to the next step until we joyfully accept our present situation as part of that plan. Secondly, he maintained that we should thank and praise God always and for everything, because, to do so is to express our acceptance of something that God is permitting to happen. So to praise God for difficult situations, such as sickness or disaster, or difficulties with one's father or mother means literally that we accept its happening, as part of God's plan

2 Cf. Pat Collins, C.M. "Overcoming Feelings of Injustice and Hurt," in *He Has Anointed Me* (Luton: New Life, 2005), 140-153.
3 *Sadhana: A Way to God* (Gujarat: Anand Press, 1978), 131.
4 *Prison to Praise* (Charisma Books, 1972); *Power in Praise* (Escondido CA: Carothers, 1980).

to reveal divine love to us. Thirdly, he referred to a quotation from 18th century Anglican clergyman William Law, "If anyone would tell you the shortest, surest way to all happiness and perfection, he must tell you to make it a rule to yourself to thank and praise God for everything that happens to you. For it is certain that *whatever seeming calamity happens to you*, if you thank and praise God for it, you will turn it into a blessing."[5] Carothers added by way of conclusion that, the very act of thanking and offering praise releases the power of God into the painful circumstances and enables God to change them. Although Carothers stressed the fact that praise and thanksgiving should be offered in obedience to God's word without any expectation of a practical advantage, he testified that he had repeatedly seen difficult and even impossible situations being transformed when God was thanked and praised in an unconditional way.

Forgiveness

Secondly, while it is true that divine forgiveness is freely available to us sinners at all times, we can only experience it to the extent that we are willing to extend it, with no strings attached, to those who have hurt or injured us. The scriptures make this abundantly clear. For instance, in Lk 6:36-39 Jesus says, "Do not judge and you will not be judged; do not condemn and you will not be condemned. Forgive and you will be forgiven... for the measure you give will be the measure you will get back." Willingness to forgive is God's way forward into Christian peace. As Bernard Meltzer, a Jewish radio host in the USA said, "When you forgive, you in no way change the past – but you sure do change the future." At this point the wounded person might like to make use of a prayer in Appendix two which was written by the late Fr Robert de Grandis who I had the pleasure of meeting many years ago.

---

5   *A Serious Call To a Devout and Holy Life*, chapt., XXII.

Receiving healing prayer for the father or mother wound

Thirdly, when the person has gained some emotional insight he or she could ask a competant person/s for prayer for what is variously called, the healing of memories, or inner healing of the father/ mother wound. I had a powerful experience of this kind of healing a number of years ago. I had been speaking and ministering at a conference somewhere in England. When we got to the end of a healing service I was feeling very tired and looking forward to relaxing in my room. As I was about to leave the auditorium two lay people approached me and asked, "Well Father, would you like a prayer of healing for yourself?" Deep down I didn't, but I had no desire to be abrupt or ungrateful, so I said a reluctant, "O.K." while hoping the prayer would be brief. Then they said, "well, have you anything in mind that you want prayer for." I hadn't thought of anything, but again to keep them happy I said, "my relationship with my mother wasn't very good, perhaps you would pray about that." Then the two lay people, a man and a woman, laid hands on me and began to pray.

As they did so I got a shock. Suddenly, and unexpectedly I had a vivid image of my father standing in front of me. Then he began to speak. "Pat" he said, "you were an exceptional boy. I can't say that I really understood you. You were too imaginative and creative for me, so I didn't know how to affirm and encourage you. I feel I let you down. I fear that you may have gotten the false impression that I didn't love you. I want to tell you, here and now, that I did really love you, but I didn't know how to express that love. I want to ask you, can you forgive me?" I was really taken aback. There was a lot of truth in what my father said. He was very different from me, quiet and uncommunicative. Because I didn't feel affirmed by him I had switched my hope for approval to my mother. She was unable to give me what I needed because of unresolved problems of her own. I felt so hurt, disappointed and resentful that it caused a good deal of conflict in our relationship. But when my father asked for my forgiveness, I felt great love for him, and said with tears in my eyes, "Of course I forgive you daddy!"

That was a significant moment of inner healing and enlightenment in my life. In a roundabout way the prayer for healing of the relationship with my mother had also been answered. I finally realised that I had switched my need for my father's male approval and affirmation to her. Once the problem with my father was healed, so, in many ways, was the relationship with my mother. In retrospect I can see how that healing of my relationship with my parents has had a positive knock on effect on my relationship with my heavenly Father. As Mal 4:6 says, "And he will turn the hearts of the fathers to their children, and the hearts of the children to their fathers." All of us can, and should, experience healing of this kind. While there are common elements, e.g., the need to forgive, the nuances will be different for each one of us.

Conclusion

As the father/mother wound is progressively healed, negative images of God are likely to be replaced by more positive ones. We grow in loving relationship with Abba Father, and come to trust in his benevolent love, more and more. As we do, scripture verses take on a new depth of life, and meaning. When I experienced healing of the father wound a number of years ago, I can remember reading the parable of the Prodigal Son with greater understanding. When I got to the words the father spoke to the elder brother, "all I have is yours" (Lk 15:31), they suddenly became alive with relevance and meaning. I sensed that God the Father was saying to me, and by extension to all his adopted children, that he would not withhold any of his many blessings from me. As this truth has made its home in my heart, a number of associated texts have become meaningful in a new way. For instance, Jesus once said, "If you, then, though you are evil [i.e. sinful], know how to give good gifts to your children, how much more will your Father in heaven give good gifts to those who ask him!" (Mt 7:11). St Paul had this same truth in mind when he wrote in Rom 8:32-33, "He who did not spare his own Son, but gave him up for us all - how will he not also, along with him, graciously give us all things?" I have discovered that my new found awareness of the benevolence and generosity of God the Father has increased my confidence in his gifts and promises. Thankfully one of the precious gifts that is being offered and one of the great promises being fulfilled is that of healing.

....

CHAPTER FOURTEEN

PRAYING FOR PHYSICAL HEALING

When one reads the gospels it would seem that most of the healings that Jesus performed were physical. For example, as was noted in chapter one, when John sent messengers to ask if Jesus was truly the promised Messiah, he replied, "Go and tell John the things which you hear and see: The blind see and the lame walk; the lepers are cleansed and the deaf hear; the dead are raised up" (Mt 11:4-5). Notice, that Jesus only referred to physical healings. Furthermore when Jesus commissioned his disciples to evangelise, he stressed the importance of physical healing. Having chosen them we are told that Jesus, "sent them out to proclaim the kingdom of God and to perform healing" (Lk 9:2). In Lk 9:6 we are told that the apostles, "began going throughout the villages, preaching the gospel and healing everywhere." Finally, before his ascension to his Father, Jesus spoke about one of four powers which would be granted to evangelists, "They will lay their hands on the sick, and they will recover" (Mk 16:18).

In these verses the emphasis is mainly on physical healing as a sign of the coming of the kingdom of God, i.e., the curse of sin has been lifted and its effects, such as illness, are being removed. Healing is the Good News in action – this was not only true for Jesus and the apostles, it can be true for us as evangelisers nowadays. God is bringing in a new world, where evil is being overcome and all sickness is beginning to be abolished, as a first instalment or intimation of the complete healing and restoration that awaits us in the second coming of Jesus. We have to demonstrate this truth by healing the sick today.

Discernment

We need to pray a silent prayer for discernment when anyone comes to us asking for prayer for physical healing. In chapter two, we spoke about two categories of illness. Firstly, there are psychosomatic ones, i.e., where the troubled mind causes disease in the body. Secondly, there are problems which are pneuma-psychosomatic in origin, i.e., where the hurting soul of the person impinges in a negative way on his or her mind and body. So when a person asks for physical healing, their illness may only be the presenting problem. The root of the person's ailment may be psychological and/or spiritual. For instance, I have noticed that stomach and colon problems are sometimes connected with repressed anger. The Holy Spirit can give us an inspiration that this may be the case. As a result, prayer for spiritual or psychological healing may be required as a prelude to prayer for physical healing.

The role of pharmacists and doctors in healing

The Old Testament confirms the dictates of common sense when it says that healing begins with doctors and pharmacists who use their natural knowledge, skills and resources in order to heal. My late father, a veterinary surgeon, used to say that, while doctors and vets like himself, are instrumental in facilitating healing of the body, ultimately it is God who heals by means of the immune system and the natural restorative powers of the body and mind. Sirach 38:1-14 endorses this attitude when it says, "Honour doctors for their services, for the Lord created them; for their gift of healing comes from the Most High... The Lord created medicines out of the earth, and the sensible will not despise them... By them the doctor heals and takes away pain; the pharmacist makes a mixture from them... My child, when you are ill, do not delay, but pray to the Lord, and he will heal you... Give the doctor his place, for the Lord created him; do not let him leave you, for you need him. There may come a time when recovery lies in the hands of physicians, for they too pray to the Lord that he grant them success in diagnosis and in healing, for the sake of preserving life." The following quotation, which is attributed to St Ignatius of Loyola, encapsulates Ben Sirach's conception of healing, "Pray as though everything depends on God; act as though everything depends on you."

The need for compassion

Time and time again we are told that when Jesus encountered those who needed physical healing he felt compassion for them. The word in Greek is *splanchnizomai*.[1] It is derived from the word *splangchna* which refers to the entrails, bowels or guts. They were thought to be the source of the most intense human feelings. So when the gospels speak of Christian compassion they are using a word that connotes, loving kindness and empathy of an intense sort for those who suffer. When we contemplate the compassion of Jesus we are contemplating the compassion of God. As Henri Nouwen has written: "When Jesus was moved to compassion, the source of all life trembled, the ground of all love burst open, and the abyss of God's immense, inexhaustible and unfathomable tenderness revealed itself."[2] We need to pray for compassion in the form of empathy like this, "Lord Jesus you told us that the teaching of the law and the prophets can be summed up in the words, "in everything, do to others what you would have them do to you'" (Mt 7:12). Grant me two gifts, the kind of love that wants what is best for others, and the kind of empathy which not only senses in an understanding way what other people are experiencing but also the ability to respond to their sufferings with sensitivity in emotional and practical ways such as healing. Amen."

When Jesus met people who needed healing he sometimes felt indignant against the ailment. In Mark 1:40-45 there is the case of the leper who came to Jesus saying, "If you are willing, you can make me clean." We are told that the response of Jesus in an earlier version

1   William Barclay, *New Testament Words* (Louisville: Westminster John Knox Press, 1974), 276-280.
2   Nouwen, Mc Neill, Morrison, *Compassion* (London: Darton, Longman & Todd, 1982), 17.

of Mark's Gospel was, "Jesus was indignant." He reached out his hand and touched the man. 'I am willing,' he said. 'Be clean!" It would seem that Jesus was angry, not with the leper, but with the leprosy. His attitude was, "how dare you spoil this man's life." I suspect that ultimately he associated a disease like leprosy with the activity of the evil one. Because he had compassion for the leper he wanted to rid him of the suffering and it's causes.

Over the years I have found that there have been occasions when I have experienced myself sharing in the indignant compassion of Jesus when confronted with the many forms of illness, disease and disability which spoil people's quality of life. Occasionally I feel confident that the indignant compassion which informs my desire to see the person being healed is a share in God's disposition and therefore an expression of the divine will for them. As a consequence, I feel assured that I will be empowered to pray effectively for them as Phil 2:13 promises. At times like these, a healer may feel that energy is flowing down his or her arms into the person, or he or she may even experience heat in the palms of the hands.

Praying in a Spirit of Peace

Physical healing has to be conducted within a context of peace. So healers try to be as relaxed as possible when praying. They encourage the person who is being prayed with, to be relaxed also. There is no need for anxious effort. The Lord says to healers, "the battle is not yours but mine" (2 Chron 20:15). Indeed, research has shown that the brainwaves of many healers change from alpha rhythms, i.e., of 14-20 cycles per second, to the beta rhythms characteristic of the sleeping state, i.e., 4-7 cycles per second. The slower brainwaves are contagious in the sense that, often those of the person being prayed with, will also change in sympathy to beta rhythms.[3] It is within this context of peace that the healer is more inclined to be open to divine inspiration, such as an appropriate scripture text, an image, a word of knowledge, or discernment of

3   Cf. Robert Eagle, *Guide to Alternative Medicine* (London: BBC, 1980), 17.

spirits. As far as the client is concerned, he or she will be more receptive to the healing activity of the Holy Spirit.

The Role of Imagination

Many healers, such as Agnes Sanford and Francis McNutt, stressed the role of using one's imagination when praying for healing. They encouraged the healer to see the afflicted part of the body being touched by the light of the Spirit. For example, when I visited Nagoya in Japan, I conducted a healing service in a Catholic University. I had received a word of knowledge about a middle-aged woman, dressed in black who had a bad hip problem. When I mentioned the ailment a woman raised her hand. I found that one of her legs was a few inches shorter than the other. While I was praying for her, I imagined that her leg was like rubber and stretching to its proper length as we prayed. When the prayer was completed we were all amazed to find that both legs were equal in length. When I returned to Japan a year later, I found that the woman was Korean and that she had truly been healed and was walking normally.

On another occasion when I was conducting a healing service for a large congregation in the Church of the Immaculate Heart of Mary in Singapore, I got a word of knowledge that there was a man present who had something seriously wrong with his liver. When I mentioned the problem a man put up his hand and I said a prayer for him from the altar. When the service ended he came into the sacristy and shared more information about his complaint. I prayed for him with the laying on of hands while imagining that his liver was flooded with the healing light of the Spirit. About a month after returning to Ireland, I received an email from the parishioner to say that when he went for a regular check-up in hospital, it was confirmed that his liver had been healed.

I can recall my father, telling me many years ago about the wonders of the body's immune system, the wonderful ability it possesses which enables it to defend itself from infections, illnesses and diseases. When people are sick, often their malady is due to the fact that their immune system has been weakened. When praying in an imaginative way, it is good to visualize the immune system being assisted by the Holy Spirit, the Lord and Giver of life, in order that it might be empowered to fight back against ailments, such as arthritis and liver disease. The body also possesses an amazing God-given ability to heal itself, e.g., when operated on by a doctor, over a period of time. When we are praying for healing we can affirm in faith that God has not only given the body an inbuilt ability to heal itself but also that the Holy Spirit is encouraging, strengthening and empowering a rapid recovery.

Conclusion

If a person feels that they have been healed, e.g., because all sense of pain has ceased, one has to be cautious about claiming that a healing has taken place. If the placebo effect, which is purely psychological, is at work, pain may be suppressed for a time by the secretion of natural opiates such as endorphins and enkephalins in the brain, but it will return. So wait for about two weeks before making a claim that a genuine healing has occurred. If possible, it is good to get the healing confirmed by a doctor. Furthermore, a person who thinks that he/she has been healed would be ill advised to stop taking medication until a doctor says it is O.K. to do so. Then it is good to edify the faith of others by telling them about the healing. As Tobit 12:7 says, "A king's secret should be kept secret, but one must declare the works of God and give thanks with due honour." That said, it is important not to exaggerate. If you do, you could bring the charism of healing into disrepute.

....

CHAPTER FIFTEEN

EXPECTANT FAITH AND HEALING

When one reads the New Testament it is obvious that faith is indispensable in healing. That said, we need to be clear about what we mean when we use the word. It was noted in chapter three that there are many interlocking forms of faith.

1) There is *deistic* faith, a belief that God exists.

2) There is *doctrinal* faith, giving mental and volitional assent to dogmas, e.g., the Nicene Creed.

3) There is *justifying* faith, which is necessary for salvation. As St Paul said in Eph 2:8-9, "For by grace you have been saved through faith. And this is not your own doing; it is the gift of God, not a result of works, so that no one may boast."

4) There is *trusting* faith which not only invests confidence in God but also in the divine providential plan and provision. Christians express that kind of faith when they believe, as St Paul said, "we know that in all things God works for the good of those who love him, who have been called according to his purpose" (Rm 8:28).

5) There is *expectant* faith, which is an intense sense of trusting faith, which is so confident in the God of the promises, and the promises of God in a particular situation of need, that it expects God to act.

In this context it is worth quoting something St Cyril of Jerusalem (313-386) said in one of his catechetical sermons. "The one word "faith" can have two meanings. One kind of faith concerns doctrines. It involves the soul's ascent to and acceptance of some particular matter. It also concerns the soul's good according to the words of the Lord, "Whoever hears my voice and believes in him who sent me has eternal life, and will not come to be judged. And again, he who believes in the Son is not condemned, but has passed from death to life"... The other kind of faith is given by Christ by means of a special grace. To one, wise sayings are given through the Spirit, to another perceptive comments by the same Spirit, to another faith by the same Spirit, to another gifts of healing. Now this kind of faith, given by the Spirit as a special favour, is not confined to doctrinal matters, for it produces effects beyond any human capability. If a person who has this faith says to this mountain move from here to there, it will move. For when anybody says this in faith, believing it will happen and having no doubt in his heart, he then receives that grace."[1]

The attitude of Jesus to faith

It has often occurred to me when reading the gospels, that it was usually the charism of expectant faith that Jesus commended in the lives of the people he met. For example, when the Roman centurion asked Jesus to help his dying servant, he showed remarkable faith of an expectant kind when he said, "Lord I am not worthy to have you come under my roof, but only say the word and my servant *will be healed*." Jesus was so impressed by the soldier's unquestioning confidence in his ability to heal, that he exclaimed: "Truly, I tell you, in no one in Israel have I found such faith" (Mt 10:10).

On more than one occasion, Jesus admonished the apostles for their lack of this kind of expectant faith. For example, when the storm blew up on the lake, the apostles were scared of sinking. They roused their sleeping companion, "Lord, save us!" they cried, "we are perishing!" (Mt 8:25). With magisterial authority, Jesus calmed the sea with a word, and turning to the apostles he said, "Why

---

1   *Cat.5, De fide et Symbolo, 10-11; PG 33, 518-519.*

are you afraid, *you of little faith?*" Having first relied on their own unsuccessful efforts to bail out the boat, they turned to Jesus with fearful and hesitant trust. He was not impressed by their level of faith. Evidently he either expected them to have such confidence in God that they themselves would have been able to say to the wind and the waves, "In the name of God, be still, be calm" (cf. Ps 107:25-30) or that they would have felt confident that they would survive the storm because Jesus was in the boat. As Is 41:10 says, "fear not, for I am with you; be not dismayed, for I am your God; I will strengthen you, I will help you."

Jesus on Unhesitating Faith

Jesus also spoke about the nature and need of charismatic faith. For example, when the apostles failed to exorcise a young boy by ridding him of an evil spirit, they asked: "Why could we not cast it out?" to which Jesus replied, "Because of your little faith. For truly, I tell you, if you have faith the size of a mustard seed, you will say to this mountain, 'Move from here to there,' and it will move; and nothing will be impossible for you" (Mt 17:19-22). When Jesus declared that all that was needed was, "Faith the size of a mustard seed" – what he meant was that a small amount of the genuine article would be enough. On another occasion Jesus cursed a fig tree which had failed to bear fruit. The following morning when Peter drew his attention to the fact that the tree had withered overnight, the Lord replied, "Have faith in God." Then he went on to say, "Truly, I tell you, if you say to this mountain, 'Be taken up and thrown into the sea,' and do not doubt in your heart, but believe that what you say will come to pass, it will be done for you. So I tell you, whatever you ask for in prayer, believe that you have received it, and it will be yours" (Mk 11:22-25).

This is a remarkable promise! Jesus says to us, the members of the Christian community of today, that we also need to have this kind of faith. In the extract from Mark eleven above, Jesus was not talking about physical mountains. What he was saying was, if there are obstacles to the coming of the kingdom, and you do not doubt in your heart (note, he does not say 'in your head'), then 'it will be done for you' and the obstacles will be removed.

Belief versus Unhesitating Faith

A person with intellectual trust accepts God's promises at a notional level, believing them to be true. However, when faced by a particular problem such as an illness, he or she may not be quite sure whether God is acting or about to act, in these particular circumstances. So, the person prays a prayer of petition in the hope that God may do something in the future, if what is asked is in accordance with the divine will, e.g., "Lord I know that nothing is impossible to you. I ask you, if it is your will, to heal this person whom you love." This is praying with hope and not with faith. Remember, Jesus never said to anyone, "your hope has made you well." Once again, recall that belief is in the head and faith in the heart.

A person with real expectant faith accepts that the promises of God are true at a notional level. But as a result of a divine revelation in a particular situation of need, e.g., a word of knowledge, he or she has no lingering doubts about the promises of God (cf. 1 Jn 5:14-16), and confidently believes that the Lord is acting, or soon will act. Often such a person prays a declaratory prayer of command rather than a supplicatory prayer of petition (Mk 11:23; Lk 17:6). Instead of having to see evidence in order to believe, this kind of confident faith believes in order to see. As the letter to the Hebrews 11:1 puts it: "Faith is the assurance (in the present) of things hoped for (in the future), the conviction (in the present) of things not seen (in the future)."

Expectant Faith Defined

In my book *Expectant Faith,* I defined the charism of faith as "a special grace, given to some believers, by the Holy Spirit, which enables them in particular situations, to discern with convinced and expectant faith of a heartfelt kind, that God will manifest his unconditional mercy and love as a sign of the coming of the

Kingdom, through a deed of power, such as a healing, exorcism or miracle."[2] The gift is evoked by a conscious awareness of God and God's will which can be revealed in one or other of many ways, but especially by the charisms of revelation, e.g., a word of knowledge. Writing about this important point, Christopher Marshall has observed in *Faith as a Theme in Mark's Narrative*, "The exertion of God's transcendent power, which faith seeks, is always subject to the constraint of God's will. The certainty of faith, in other words, presupposes revelatory insight into the divine intention, though this must be actualized by the believer's volitional commitment to refuse doubt and seek undivided faith (cf. Mk 5:36; 9:22-24)."[3] Whatever way it comes, the revelation of God's will evokes the inner certainty that is characteristic of expectant faith. Over the years I have found that there is a spectrum of faith ranging from one to ten in intensity. Even when one's expectant faith would only merit a three out of ten, more often than not, it is sufficient, thereby confirming what Jesus said about the mustard seed of faith in Mt 17:20. One way or another, as St. Paul pointed out in Rm 10:17, "faith comes from hearing the message (*rhema*), and the message is heard through the word of Christ."

A Personal Testimony

In the 1970s I was prayerfully wrestling with a passage in Mk 11:20-23 about mountain moving faith. Around the same time, a pupil of mine, a fine footballer, injured his back. He was in considerable pain, found it hard to sleep or study, and was unable to play on the College team. It had reached the semi-finals of the MacRory Cup that particular year. At one point a number of the sixth formers approached me. "Father, we need Neil for the cup match," they said, "we have heard you preaching about God's willingness to answer prayer. Will you pray for him?" I said I'd consider it, if

2   Pat Collins, C.M., *Expectant Faith and the Power of God* (Dublin: Columba, 1998), 49.
3   (Cambridge: Cambridge University Press, 1994), 168.

Neil asked me himself. Secretly I was hoping he wouldn't. Then the headmaster approached me and made a similar request. I gave him the same evasive answer that I had already given to the boys.

Finally, Neil himself came to see me and requested prayer. I arranged to meet him after school. When we got together I read the passage from Mark 11:20-23. "Do you believe what the Lord promises?" I asked. "Well, let's put it this way, Father, I believe that what the Lord says is true, but I find it hard to believe it will be true in my case." "I'm much the same," I said, "but we will pray and see what happens." I put my hands on Neil's back while imagining that the light of God's healing love was shining upon it and within it. As my concentration deepened, I found myself telling the injury to yield to the power of God at work in all the cells. As I was doing this I became convinced that what we were praying for was being granted. I concluded by thanking the Lord for what he was doing and would continue to do in Neil's back. When the prayer was over I asked Neil how he felt. "To tell the truth, Father, the pain is worse now!" "Take no notice," I said, "Imitate St Peter when he was walking on the water. Keep your mind on Jesus; forget about your symptoms. We were praying for a healing, not a miracle. It is a process; it will take time."

When I returned to my room I stormed heaven. "Don't let me down Lord," I prayed, half joking and whole in earnest, "otherwise your reputation and mine will be in ruins in this school." I must admit that the following morning my faith levels were weakening. When I got into class I asked Neil in a whisper how he was. "I had a great night's sleep," he said cheerily, "for the first time since the accident. My back is fine now," and he did a number of twists and bends to prove the point. That was the first time I saw my faith lead to healing.

Conclusion

We conclude this chapter with some words of Kathryn Kulhman, "Faith is more than belief. It is more than confidence. It is more than trust. It is more than the sum total of these things... Faith as God himself imparts it to the heart, is spiritual. It's warm. It's vital. It lives. It throbs. Its power is absolutely irresistible when it is imparted to the heart by the Lord... Heart belief is faith. Mind belief is nothing more than deep desire combined with mental assent." [4] Lord we believe, help our unbelief (cf. Mk 9:24).

4   Jamie Buckingham, *A Glimpse into Glory*, (Los Angeles: Bridge Publishing Inc, 1983), 45.

....

CHAPTER SIXTEEN

GROWING IN EXPECTANT FAITH

In chapter fourteen we noted how important expectant faith is where healing and miracle working are concerned. In 1 Cor 14:1 St Paul said, "Let love be your highest goal! But you should also desire the special abilities the Spirit gives." So while the gift of faith is a gratuitous one, the community is encouraged to desire it like the other gifts. Not everyone receives the charism of faith, but they pray that it will be given to some of the members of the community or group. This raises the question, is there anything that the members of the community can do, in order to receive the charism of expectant faith and to grow in that type of mountain-moving trust. We will look at a number of things that can be done.

Build on the Virtue of Faith

St Cyril of Jerusalem who was referred to in a previous chapter, said, "As far as it depends on you, cherish saving faith, which leads you to God, and you will receive the higher gift, i.e., the charism of faith, which no effort of yours can reach, no powers of yours attain."[1] Cyril seemed to be saying that if we have strong faith in Jesus as our Saviour, that will be a stepping stone to the charism of faith. The closer we get to Christ, the more we will trust him, and that will prepare us, if God so wishes, to graduate to the gift of expectant faith.

We are enabled to grow in the virtue of faith by confessing un-repented sin to God and believing that, for those who are in

---

1   *Cat.5, De fide et Symbolo, 10-11; PG 33, 518-519.*

Christ Jesus as a result of baptism and personal faith, "there is now no condemnation" (Rm 8:1). Justifying faith is also nourished by means of daily prayer, scripture reading and reception of the sacraments. As a result, one grows to have an ever-deepening knowledge of Christ and the power of his resurrection at work in one's life. This kind of faith relationship, gives rise to an increasing, and unimpeded awareness, born of trust, that God, "is able to do far more abundantly than all that we ask or think, according to the power at work within us" (Eph 3:20). Speaking of that inner power, Paul said, "it is the same as the mighty strength which God the Father used when he raised Christ from death and seated him at his right side in the heavenly world" (Eph 1:19-20). While normally Christian discipleship involves a faithful and persevering following of Christ and his love in the humdrum circumstances of everyday life, occasionally it may involve a manifestation of the power of God, e.g., in the form of a healing or miracle. What St Cyril was asserting was that there is a continuity between one kind of faith and the other.

The Example of Men and Women of Faith

Another way of growing in charismatic faith is to become associated, directly or indirectly, with people who exercise this gift. For example, many people have testified to the fact that their growth in charismatic faith was greatly helped when they attended a healing service conducted by a well-known healer, e.g., Fr Peter Rookey, Damian Stayne, Eddie Stones, or Sr. Briege McKenna, etc. For instance, in his book *Growing in Faith*, Steve Clark says that in the late nineteen sixties or early seventies he saw many people being cured by the late Kathryn Kuhlman at one of her 'miracle services' in the 7,000 seat Shrine Auditorium in Los Angeles. He reported that at one point, "people started coming up to the stage, and they told about the different things that had happened to them. One was cured of arthritis, someone else came up with his crutches to report on his cure, a boy deaf in one ear could hear with it. Dozens of people came forward with impressive healings."[2] Later in the book, Clark observed, "because I saw what God *could* do, I found it easier to believe in what he *would* do."[3] Not all of us have had the opportunity of witnessing the ministry of such a gifted Charismatic as Kathryn Kulhman. But we can read about their lives, study their writings and watch relevant videos when they are available.

For example, I have found that inspiring biographies and books of testimony to do with Kathryn Kuhlman's life and ministry have been a great inspiration. There is a wonderful biography of Kathryn, *Daughter of Destiny* by Jamie Buckingham. There are also three books by Kathryn containing awesome healing testimonies, *Nothing is Impossible with God; I Believe in Miracles;* and *God Can Do It Again.* Like many others I have learned a great deal from the life and ministry of English Pentecostal, Smith Wigglesworth, who was renowned not only for his great faith but also his ability to heal. Many of his core teachings are contained in an anthology, *Greater Works.* Large numbers of people have been inspired by Sr. Briege McKenna's *Miracles Do Happen: God Can Do the Impossible.* People who read Damian Stayne's instructive and edifying book, *Renew your Wonders: Spiritual Gifts for Today* will find that it contains sound teaching and inspiring testimonies to do with the gift of healing. I have also discovered that there are many faith building and instructive videos on You Tube. For instance, I have been very impressed and edified by those of people like John Wimber, Shawn Bolz, Randy Clark, Todd White, Bill Johnson and Heidi Baker who are involved in charismatic types of healing ministry.

An Imaginative Spiritual Exercise

In *The Healing Light* Agnes Sanford proposed the following imaginative prayer exercise as a way of increasing faith:

- Lay aside your worries. Quieten your mind and concentrate on the presence of God.

2   (Notre Dame: Charismatic Renewal Services, 1972), 16.
3   Ibid, 41.

- Remind yourself that there is a source of life beyond your own. Get in touch with that Source of life by saying a prayer like this, "Lord of life, increase in me at this time your life-giving power."
- Believe and affirm that the power is coming into your deepest self. Recall what Jesus promised in Lk 11:13, "If you then, though you are evil, know how to give good gifts to your children, how much more will your Father in heaven give the Holy Spirit to those who ask him!"
- Accept God's power with confident trust. It becomes yours as you accept it with thanksgiving. You could say, "Thank you that your life is coming into me even now and filling me, body, mind and soul."
- Observe the operations of God's life in yours. In order to do so decide on some tangible thing that you wish to be accomplished by that power so that you will know without question that your experiment succeeded, e.g., praying that a friend's cold would be cured, that a relative would get a job etc. If you pray in the awareness that the Spirit is in you, with the passage of time you will get the grace to pray more boldly.

Here is a personal example of what I mean when I say that we have to put our faith into action. In the Autumn of 2019 I conducted a healing service in a hotel in Charleville, county Cork. Beforehand, I spent time, as is my custom, praying for God's grace and asking for guidance about the illnesses that would be healed. A number of images and ideas came to mind, but the strangest and most unlikely of all was a sense that a woman would be present who had a hole in her eye, and that it was associated with great pain. I thought to myself that I had never come across anything like that in all my years. I mentioned this condition in a hesitant way during the service and asked if anyone present suffered from it. I was amazed when a woman raised her hand. I found out afterwards that she was suffering from many health problems, one of which was a problem with her eyes which were in danger of progressively losing their sight. I cannot now remember the details. In any case, it turned out that as part of her treatment this woman had to endure the acute pain of being injected in the eye. Needless to say, that left a hole so to speak. Although she couldn't bear the thought of having to endure more injections of that kind her specialist told her they would be necessary if she wanted to retain her sight. When I found that the word of knowledge was accurate, I was convinced that her healing would be in accord with the will of God. I asked people near her to put a gentle hand on her as I prayed a prayer for her at the microphone. Since then I have discovered that the woman with the eye problem was able to confirm that her sight has been improving ever since. The other injections have been cancelled, and her overall health has gotten progressively better.

Focus on the living Word of God

Hebrews 11:1 provides us with the Bible's only definition of faith, "Now faith is confidence in what we hope for and assurance about what we do not see." It is equally surprising to find that there is only one text in the Bible which tells us how to grow in faith. It is in Rom 10:17-18 and reads, "faith comes from hearing the message, and the message is heard through the word of Christ." When a person truly hears the gospel message, and confesses with their mouth that Jesus is Lord and believes in their heart that God raised Him from the dead they will experience salvation (cf. Rm 10:9). This dynamic, however, is not just restricted to the *kerygma*, or message of salvation, it can also apply to any revelatory word from God. As Prov 4:20-22, says, "My child, be attentive to my words; incline your ear to my sayings. Let them not escape from your sight; keep them within your heart. For they are life to those who find them, *and healing to your body.*"

As one contemplates God's word in this way, it can jump off the page as a living and inspiring word for now (cf. Heb 4:12). Because it reveals God's existential will, it evokes the gift of expectant faith. I think that Smith Wigglesworth had this in mind when he said near the end of his life, "There are four principles we need to maintain: first, read the Word of God; second, consume the Word of God until it consumes you; third believe the Word of God; fourth, act on the Word."[4] It needs to be said that one can hear the word of God in many ways during prayer, e.g., as a word of knowledge which can come in the form of an image, vision, inner voice, or an intellectual understanding of God's purposes. Ps 18:30 states that, "The Lord's word is flawless," and Is 55:11 assures us that the word of God contains the God given power to fulfill what it says, "so shall my word be that goes out from my mouth; it shall not return to me empty, but it shall accomplish that which I purpose, and shall succeed in the thing for which I sent it."

Conclusion

Kathryn Kulhman once said with disarming simplicity, but great insight, "You do not pray for faith; you seek the Lord, and faith will come."[5] Kathryn said that charismatic faith is not the result of human effort. Paradoxically, it is when, we forget about ourselves and concentrate on the Lord, by means of contemplative attention, that faith is *evoked* in the heart. Kathryn said, "Look up and see Jesus! He is your faith, He is our faith. It is not faith that you must seek, but Jesus."[6] She warned that faith is often compromised, as it was for the apostles during the storm on the lake, by looking at God in the light of the problem, rather than looking at the problem in the light of heartfelt relationship with God. So focus on God and see pain and suffering in the light of that relationship.

---

4   https://www.jonasclark.com/smith-wigglesworth-the-apostle-faith/
5   *I Believe in Miracles* (London: Lakeland, 1974), 203.
6   Ibid., 204.

....

CHAPTER SEVENTEEN

DISCERNING GOD'S WILL IN HEALING

We can presume that because he knew he was the divine Son of God, Jesus realized that he had the power to heal and perform miracles. So it is very interesting to see his response to his mother's request that he do something helpful when the young couple were in danger of running out of wine at the marriage feast of Cana. We are told that, "Jesus said to her, "Woman, what concern is that to you and to me? My hour has not yet come" (Jn 2:4). While Jesus did not deny the fact that he could perform a miracle, he seemed to be saying that he didn't think it was God's will that he would do so at that particular time in those particular circumstances. He explained on another occasion, "Very truly I tell you, the Son can do nothing by himself; he can do only what he sees his Father doing" (Jn 5:19). We can infer from this statement that whenever Jesus performed a healing, he was authorised to do so because he had discerned it was the will of his Father. It has to be much the same in the lives of contemporary Christian believers.

In the light of the previous point the following words from 1 Jn 5:14-16 are important, "And this is the confidence we have in him, that if we ask anything according to his will, he hears us. And if we know that he hears us in whatever we ask, we know that we have obtained the requests made of him." Two points are important here. Firstly, from a Johannine point of view, those who want their prayers for healing to be granted, need to strive to live holy lives in accord with the commandments as encapsulated in the great command of love (cf. 1 Jn 3:23). We live by that commandment by trying, with God's help, to love others as God loves us in Christ. Secondly, prayer should not be selfish or arbitrary, but led by the Spirit and in accord with God's will (cf. Gal 5:16; Mt 6:10). Although John doesn't mention it, there is reason to pray with confidence for the gift of wisdom and its ability to reveal what God wants (cf. Is 11:2; Jm 1:5-6). Does God want me to heal the person of this particular ailment at this particular time? The answer does not come through human reasoning. Rather the Spirit reveals the answer.

We know how John declares, that if people pray in this way, not only are they heard, they have *already obtained* what they asked for. This awareness displays a remarkable degree of expectant faith, one shot through with super-eminent certainty characteristic of the charism of faith. In terms of what Jesus said in Mk 11:24, it believes that it has already received what was asked for in faith. Once again, *present certainty* is the basis of *future hope*, faith conviction in the here and now, a sure pledge of blessings to come. It seems clear that in these verses John is going beyond trusting faith of the hesitant kind, to the charism of faith of the expectant kind.

God's General and Specific Will

Anyone who is asked to pray for a sick person can be clear about God's general, active will. It is to heal people of whatever ails them. However, God's general desire will only be completely accomplished in the second coming when, as Rev 21:4 says, God "will wipe every tear from their eyes. There will be no more death or mourning or crying or pain, for the old order of things has passed away." In the meantime, the period between the Resurrection and the Second Coming of Jesus, we have to tune in to God's existential will in the here and now. So we ask, is this the *kairos* moment, God's appointed time to heal as an intimation of the inauguration of a new heavens and a new earth? *Chronos* is the Greek word for secular, sequential time 24/7, but *kairos* is sacred time, the special moment when God intervenes in a saving way. For instance, at the wedding feast of Cana, it would seem that Jesus came to see in Mary's compassionate concern, a revelation of the Father's will and therefore the *kairos* moment. So it is not surprising to find that Paul said, "we have not ceased to pray for you, asking that you may be filled with the knowledge of his will in all spiritual wisdom and understanding, so as to walk in a manner worthy of the Lord, fully pleasing to him" (Col 1:9-10). We the modern disciples of Christ have to continually tune in to the will of God if we want God's authority to heal.[1] The question is, how do we tune in to the will of God?

The Rhema Word

The word of God can be viewed as a noun or a verb. As a noun, God's *logos* word is objectively true upon the page. As such it can be studied and interpreted in an academic way. As a verb, that is spoken to the heart, the *rhema* word of God can become subjectively true, at a particular time, in a particular circumstance, for a particular individual/s. Speaking about the relationship between *logos* and *rhema* Derek Prince suggested in *Faith to Live By* that it could be expressed in the following statements:

> "*Rhema* takes the eternal — *logos* — and injects it into time.
>
> *Rhema* takes the heavenly — *logos* — and brings it down to earth.
>
> *Rhema* takes the potential — *logos* — and makes it actual.
>
> *Rhema* takes the general — *logos* — and makes it specific.
>
> Rhema takes a portion of the total — *logos* — and presents it in a form that a man can assimilate."[2]

1   Cf. Pat Collins, C.M. *Guided by God: Ordinary and Charismatic Ways of Discovering God's Will* (Luton: New Life, 2015).

2   https://www.charismamag.com/anniversary/pages-from-our-past/24027-derek-prince-faith-to-live-by

God can guide us by means of a *rhema* word that jumps alive off the page, (e.g., as one engages in *Lectio Divina*),[3] with relevance and meaning, into the heart. Deut 29:29 says, "The secret things belong to the Lord our God, but the things revealed belong to us." Ps 119:105 adds, "Your word is a lamp for my feet, a light on my path." We are told that such a word will be empowered to achieve its divinely intended purpose. For instance we read that, "The Lord was with Samuel as he grew up, and he let none of Samuel's words fall to the ground" (1 Sam 3:19), in other words they all bore fruit.

An Inspiration

St Vincent de Paul once said, "There is another way of knowing God's will, and it is by inspiration: for often he enlightens our understanding and gives impulses to our heart to be inspired by his will."[4] This can happen when you are praying with great compassion for someone and as you ardently desire his or her healing, you suddenly realise that you are sharing in Christ's compassion and desire. That being so, you get the inner conviction that it is the Lord's will to heal the person right now. I can recall this happening when praying for an epileptic boy who had been brought to me by his uncle and aunt. Their love was quite apparent in the ardent desire they so clearly had that he would be helped. I felt my compassion was a small share in Christ's compassion and was therefore convinced that he would be healed. So I laid hands on his head and prayed for him. I was told sometime later by the uncle and aunt that he had experienced no more *petit* or *grand-mal* attacks.

A Dream or a Vision

The Lord can guide us by means of Spirit-prompted dreams and visions. As Job 33:14-15 says: "For God does speak - now one way,

3   On *Lectio Divina* (divine reading) see Benedict XVI apostolic exhortation *Verbum Domini* (The word of the Lord), pars 86-87.
4   *Correspondence, Conferences, Documents*, Vol. 12 (New York: New City Press, 2009), 133.

now another - though man may not perceive it. In a dream, in a vision of the night." God's existential will is revealed to some people by means of a night-time vision. More commonly people may receive a vision as a sort of day dream by means of which God can reveal the divine will, with or without explanatory words. When I'm preparing for healing services, I sometimes receive guidance in this way. I will see the person, sometimes where they are sitting and know what is wrong with them. A few years ago in London, I saw a woman in my mind's eye. When I asked the Lord what was wrong with her, I had the impression that she suffered from an ingrown eyelash problem (trichiasis). I thought it was unlikely to be a true word from the Lord because I'd never heard of such a condition. During the healing service I did ask if any woman suffered from that problem. A hand went up. We prayed for her. The next day she was able to report that she had been healed. As a result she was able to cancel having a hospital procedure to correct the problem.

A Word of Knowledge

The word of knowledge says David Pytches, is a "supernatural revelation of facts about a person or situation, which is not learned through the efforts of the natural mind." One can hear an inner voice speaking and giving guidance. It is similar to seeing a dream or vision. It is as if a voice other than one's own is speaking to you. I have often received this kind of guidance. This happened a few years ago when I was ministering in Leeds Cathedral. I knew that a man would come who suffered from repeated nightmares. In spite of asking God to remove them on numerous occasions he would still be suffering from them. I felt the Lord was saying they were due to the influence of an evil spirit. When people came forward for the anointing I ministered to them without any conversation. But when I came to one man I felt compelled to ask him why he wanted the anointing. He said that he been suffering for many years from terrible nightmares. Although he had often asked God to remove them, nothing had happened. I could see that what he said confirmed the accuracy of the word of knowledge I had received in prayer. I assured him that the Lord would help him and that he needed to be delivered from an evil spirit. I anointed him with expectant faith and felt a real impartation of the Spirit as I did so. Although I have never met him since, I was amazed at the way in which the Lord revealed the man's problem to me a few hours before meeting him.

Some time ago I led a healing service in a town on the North coast of Sicily. During one of my talks, it suddenly occurred to me that an elderly woman was present who had pain running across her back on the left-hand side. I stopped speaking and asked if there was anyone present with those symptoms. A woman put up her hand and said that she was suffering from shingles and that her symptoms were just as I had described. I said a quick prayer and continued my talk. The next day the woman was able to report that all her pain had disappeared.

A few years ago I led a healing service in Kilkenny. At one point I felt that God was telling me that a woman was present who suffered from bad headaches. Then I was given to understand that her condition was related to her periods. Then the name of a medical condition came into my mind. I could not pronounce it properly and I had no idea what it referred to. When I struggled to enunciate what it was, a doctor who was present said that the word was endometriosis while explaining that it was a problem of the womb. When I asked if any woman present was suffering from those symptoms, immediately, a lady put up her hand and we prayed for her. After Christmas, I received a card which contained the following message, "I had asked the Lord to heal me during the service. You said you hadn't heard this in a long time but there was somebody in the room suffering from headaches relating to her periods and endometriosis. I am overjoyed to say – all of my symptoms have disappeared - and I constantly praise the Lord."

Praying within One's Measure of Faith

In Rm 12:3 we read, "think of yourself with sober judgment, in accordance with the faith God has distributed to each of you." Although I'm aware that I am taking the phrase "with the faith God has distributed to each of you," out of its context, nevertheless it can be applied to prayer for healing. We need to pray within the measure of faith we have received whether trusting or expectant. I have often found that I begin such a prayer with trusting faith. In those circumstances, I will pray in a general, non-specific way like this, "Lord you are the God of love, I know that you love (name) and because you love him/her you want what is best for him/her. I thank you that your love is even now at work carrying out your will of peace. I thank you that your Spirit is at work in all the cells that need your help while revealing your will and enabling them to respond."

Notice that while this prayer is true it is also vague and fairly non-specific. However I have found that as I push my trusting faith to the limit, it sometimes morphs into expectant faith as I sense that God is at work in a specific way. It may be, that as I pray I might get a revelation, in any of the ways already described. As I receive that new measure of faith I can pray in a more authoritative way by means of the prayer of command, e.g., "I command the ailing cells, be healed in the name of the Lord Jesus, and I thank you God, that even now that healing has begun."

Conclusion

When we pray for healing we need to tune in to God's will as best we can. We also have to avoid the kind of presumption that would lead us to pray beyond the measure of faith we have received. Sometimes in such a situation the praying person moves from a general prayer of petition to a more specific prayer of command. Finally, as was mentioned already, it is important not to make premature claims about a healing. Because of the well-attested influence of the placebo effect, which may suppress pain for a few days, we have to wait to see whether the improvement is long-lasting or not.

Chapter Eighteen

....

Healing and the Anointing of the Sick

The practice of anointing the sick had its roots in the Gospels. In Mk 6:13 we are told that, "They went out and preached that people should repent. They drove out many demons and anointed many sick people with oil and healed them." The oil was the outward sign of the inner gift of God's healing unction. In the New Testament Church there was also a link between anointing and healing, "Is anyone among you sick? Let them call the elders of the church to pray over them and anoint them with oil in the name of the Lord. And the prayer offered in faith will make the sick person well; the Lord will raise them up. If they have sinned, they will be forgiven" (Jm 5:14-15).

At first charismatic forms of healing predominated in the early Church. However, within a generation or two healing was institutionalised when it became the domain of bishops and priests in and through sacramental anointing. Scripture scholars such as Martin Dibelius, Richard Kugelman and Charles Gusmer stress the fact that in the letter of James sick people were not sending for lay people with a charismatic gift of healing, but rather for ordained office holders in the church. Martin Dibelius wrote, "If this passage were speaking about pneumatics in possession of a charisma, or spiritual gift, then it would be calling for the "charismatic" gift of healing, as it is mentioned in 1 Cor 12:9; 28; 30. But instead, the reference is to the elders of the church. They must be the bearers of the miraculous power by virtue of the fact that they are elders, for otherwise why would they be called upon and not others?... Their healing power must be connected with their official character... We have no knowledge of a development within the Jewish community which makes an office the vehicle of strong ecstatic-pneumatic powers."[1]

James says that the prayer over the sick should be made with faith. Did he have the charism of faith, mentioned by Paul in 1 Cor 12:9, in mind? The fact that he goes on to cite the charismatic faith of Elijah in Jm 5:17-19, suggests that perhaps he had.[2] Martin Dibelius supports the belief that the prayer of faith mentioned in Jm 5:15 involves the charism of faith. He says that it, "Corresponds to the charismatic faith with which we are familiar from the stories in the Gospels, a faith which looks for an answer to prayer, even expects miracles."[3] That would mean that although the anointing of the sick was administered by a priest and not a charismatic, in so far as he needed expectant faith to be effective means that a charismatic dimension was retained in the sacrament. Although this is a debatable point, I suspect that the need for expectant faith might explain why so few sacramental anointings seem to lead to either inner or physical healing.

Whereas in the early Church the primary emphasis was on healing of the whole person, including spiritual and physical healing, in later centuries that emphasis shifted to spiritual salvation. For example, when St Jerome (340-420) translated the Bible into Latin, he used *salvo* exclusively *to* mean "to save" in order to get across the meaning of *sozien* which in Greek can be legitimately translated as "to save or to heal." Because Jerome's Vulgate version of the Bible became the official Western text, this misleading emphasis on salvation only, influenced subsequent understanding of the sacrament of anointing. Gradually the emphasis began to shift from getting

---

1 *James: A Commentary on the Epistle of James* (San Francisco: Harper Collins, 1997), 94.

2 Arnold Bittlinger cites Elijah as an exemplar of the charism of faith in *Gifts and Graces: A Commentary on 1 Corinthians 12-14* (London: Hodder & Stoughton, 1973), 32-33.

3 James, op. cit., 254.

better from illness to preparation for death. The Council of Trent (1545-1563) reinforced this lopsided understanding.

Speaking about the sacrament of the anointing of the sick, the Council of Trent stated, "This anointing is to be administered to the sick, especially to those who are so dangerously ill that they may seem close to death." Not surprisingly, in the period from Trent until the Second Vatican Council, the anointing of the sick was seen mainly as a way of preparing people spiritually, who were in danger of death. *De facto* prayer for physical healing was largely ignored. As a result, those who desired to be healed had to resort to private prayer, relics of the saints, holy wells, or go on pilgrimage to shrines such as Lourdes, where healings were known to occur.

Vatican II Reform

Happily, all this began to change in recent years.

- Firstly, the fathers of Vatican II modified the scholastic and Tridentine understanding of the sacrament. They stated that instead of being called "Extreme Unction" as heretofore, the sacrament was to be referred to as the "Anointing of the sick." Consequently, it was to be administered to those who were seriously ill, and not just to those who were dying.

- Secondly, the essential purpose of the sacrament was changed. Instead of focusing attention exclusively on the forgiveness of sins and spiritual comfort, it also focused on healing of the whole person, i.e., body and mind, as well as soul. "Assistance from the Lord by the power of his Spirit is meant to lead the sick person to healing of the soul, but also of the body if such is God's will."[4]

- Thirdly, the Council fathers said that the sacrament should be administered in a communal setting where family, friends and neighbours would be able to support the sick person by their faith-filled prayers. They stated, "The sick

---

4   *Catechism of the Catholic Church*, par. 1520.

should prepare themselves to receive it (the sacrament) with good dispositions, assisted by their pastor and the whole ecclesial community, which is invited to surround the sick in a special way through their prayers and fraternal attention. "[5] The community prays for this person and the priest acts on behalf of the community. Surely the most important disposition of the recipient, is that of faith. Ideally it would be a faith that is informed with God-given wisdom and expectancy. It would know that God *is* going to "save" and to "raise up," i.e., to comfort and to heal.

- Fourthly, the Conciliar document stresses the importance of faith-filled prayer as one of the four main elements in the celebration of the sacrament. The phrase, "faith of the Church" can have two layers of meaning. It can refer in a doctrinal way to the effects of the sacrament. It can also refer to trusting faith in God's greatness, goodness, love, etc., and in the promises of God, especially those which have to do with the Lord's willingness to answer prayer. Surely, it is this second point, in particular, that James had in mind when he spoke about the prayer of faith, i.e., charismatic faith. The people involved with the anointing, the priest, the person who is ill, and the community need trusting faith. But they need to be conscientious and pray within the "measure of faith" they have received (Rm 12:3), either trusting faith of the hesitant kind, or trusting faith of the expectant kind (i.e. the charism of faith).

A testimony

When I was part of a mission team in St Eugene's Cathedral parish in Derry, in the mid 1980s, I witnessed a memorable healing. A man approached me who had a terrible bladder complaint. He showed me a letter from his consultant informing him about the time he

---

5   *Catechism of the Catholic Church*, par. 1516

was expected in hospital to undergo corrective surgery. However, the man had a strong feeling that he should come to the mission where he hoped to be healed. Although I was feeling exhausted as the mission drew to an end, I anointed the parishioner with as much faith as I could muster. A year later I was involved in another mission in Derry when I was approached by the man I had anointed a year before. He told me that he had been completely healed and that his surgery had been cancelled. In the Autumn of 2019, I spoke at a novena in St Eugene's. While there I was approached by a lady. She asked me if I could remember anointing a man with a bad bladder complaint many years before. I said that I did. Then she told me that she was his wife. She informed me that following his anointing not only was he totally healed he never had any bladder problems from that time until his death two months previously.

Oil of Gladness

In recent years, members of the Charismatic Renewal have revived the blessing of olive oil for use for non-sacramental anointing for the healing of the sick. It is not only popular but effective when administered with loving faith by lay people. The blessing taken from the Roman Ritual is printed in full in Appendix three. Speaking of the oil of gladness a reading from the instruction to the newly-baptized at Jerusalem says, "Christ was anointed with the spiritual oil of gladness, that is with the Holy Spirit, who is called the oil of gladness because he is the author of spiritual joy; and you have been anointed with chrism because you have become fellows and sharers of Christ... It is applied to your forehead and organs of sense with a symbolic meaning; the body is anointed with visible ointment, and the soul is sanctified by the holy, hidden Spirit. While the anointing of baptism is "no mere or ordinary ointment; it is the gift of Christ, which through the presence of the Holy Spirit instils his divinity into us so subsequently, anointing with the oil of gladness, blessed for use by lay people, can grace people with inner comfort, and even healing of mind and body. As Heb 1:9 says, "God has anointed you with the oil of gladness."[6]

Whereas only priests can administer the sacrament of the anointing of the sick, lay people can use the oil of gladness as a sacramental, when praying for healing. According to par. 1670 of the *Catechism of the Catholic Church*, "Sacramentals do not confer the grace of the Holy Spirit in the way that the sacraments do, but by the Church's prayer, they prepare us to receive grace and dispose us to cooperate with it." That said, I have seen the sacrament and the sacramental both being efficacious in healing the sick.

Conclusion

Homilists and catechists need to stress the fact that the anointing of the sick is sometimes intended to bring about, not just spiritual, but also physical and mental healing, if and when, either the minister, the recipient, or some other caring person/s is graced with the charism of unhesitating faith. That said, preaching on this point has to be nuanced and sensitive. Otherwise it will create the impression that if the person's prayer is not answered it is due to his or her own lack of faith. By definition, the charism of faith, is a special gift of God which is sometimes given to some people. Good catechetical preaching, however, could explain that such faith can be evoked by means of a Spirit-given inspiration which reveals the Lord's existential will (see Rm 12:2; 1 Cor 2:15-16; Eph 1:9; Col 1:9). Expectant faith can also be evoked by powerful testimony about a healing, as a result of the anointing of the sick.

Although quite a number of people are healed having received the sacrament of the anointing of the sick, many others are not. Speaking about this anomaly par. 1521 of the *Catechism of the Catholic Church* says, "By the grace of this sacrament the sick person receives the strength and the gift of uniting himself more closely to Christ's Passion: in a certain way he is consecrated to bear fruit

---

6   *Divine Office*, Vol II, Office of Readings, Easter Octave: Friday, p. 415.

by configuration to the Saviour's redemptive Passion. Suffering, a consequence of original sin, acquires a new meaning; it becomes a participation in the saving work of Jesus." We will return to this subject in chapter twenty one.

Chapter Nineteen

....

Healing and the Eucharist

Earlier in this book we noted that when Jesus proclaimed the coming of the kingdom of God, he was saying two main things. Firstly, he announced the lifting of the curse of sin as a result of the unmerited outpouring of God's mercy and love. All they had to do to receive it was to believe in Jesus and his gracious message. Secondly, as a sign of the forgiveness of sins, Jesus removed the penalty of sin by healing the sick and driving out evil spirits. This good news was made possible because Jesus was willing, in his great love, to become a ransom for us by acting as our scapegoat on the cross. He took the curse and penalty of sin upon himself. As scripture tells us, "Christ redeemed us from the curse of the law by becoming a curse for us, for it is written: "Cursed is everyone who hangs on a tree" (Gal 3:13). Scripture also talks about Christ's removal of the penalty of sin when it says, "By his wounds you have been healed" (1Pt 2:24-25).

All of this is sacramentally present in the Mass, which makes the sacrifice of Calvary to be available in our time.[1] There is great symbolic significance in the gesture of the priest when he extends his hands over the bread and wine at the consecration. It is reminiscent of Lev 16:21-23 where we are told that a priest would

---

1   Dom Odo Casel, O.S.B. (1886-1948), a famous pre Vatican II liturgist maintained, that in the Mass, the mystery of Christ (which is Christ himself) is neither merely imitated or remembered. In liturgy, he believed, the saving deed of Christ was objectively re-presented as an efficacious reality, thus enabling believers to enter into salvific contact with it.

bring, "a live goat and laying hands upon its head, confess over it the sins of the people of Israel. He shall lay all their sins upon the head of the goat and send it into the desert." In every Mass we pray repeatedly for the lifting of the curse of sin, e.g., when we say the Confiteor, and when we say before receiving Holy Communion, "Lamb of God you take away the sin of the world, have mercy on us." In the Mass the penalty of sin, in the form of sickness, disease and disability can also be removed from us. For example, before receiving Holy Communion, we pray, "May the receiving of your body and blood, Lord Jesus Christ, not bring me to judgement and condemnation, but through your loving mercy be for me protection in mind and body and a healing remedy." I firmly believe that if we receive the Eucharist with faith it can bring about healing of soul, mind and body.

The Mass contains many other mentions of it. Quite often the liturgical readings of the day will speak about healing. That fact affords the celebrant an opportunity to give a homily on the subject of healing, its nature, and the means we have of experiencing it. Sometimes, the sacrament of the anointing of the sick is administered after the liturgy of the word. For example, anointing within the Eucharist is a common feature of Masses which are celebrated in the basilica in Knock. Frequently, the Eucharist will contain prayers which ask God for healing. For example, the Mass for the sick, in the missal, contains the following opening prayer, "All powerful and ever living God, the lasting health of all who believe in you, hear us as we ask your loving help for the sick; restore their health, that they may again offer joyful thanks in your Church. Amen."

Jesus the Poultice of God
Some time ago when I was reflecting on this mystery of salvation I recalled an occasion in my childhood when I got a nasty wound in my leg. I had been climbing a tree. A branch broke and a piece of wood stuck into my thigh muscle. As soon as I got home

my mother removed it and dressed the wound. Sometime later, my father made a poultice, which was designed to draw out any infection, while at the same time disinfecting and protecting the damaged tissues. In the event it was very effective. Then it occurred to me that in the Eucharist, Christ our scapegoat, is the poultice of God. He not only enfolds our woundedness, he absorbs the evil of our sin and sickness into himself while imparting his forgiveness and healing to us. As St Paul testified, "God made him who had no sin to be sin for us, so that in him we might become the righteousness of God" (2 Cor 5:21).

Healing and Holy Communion

It is clear that the healing power of the Eucharist is most evident in the prayers that precede holy communion. We will look at five instances. The words, "Hallowed be thy name" (Mt 6:9) in the Lord's Prayer are not primarily about what we do for God, i.e., praising his holy name, but about what God does for us, i.e., by manifesting his majesty, holiness and saving power. In Ezech 36:23 we read, "I will hallow my great name which you have profaned among the nations." God does this, pre-eminently, by ushering in his kingdom, hence the next petition, "Thy kingdom come." While these petitions refer primarily to the end times when Christ will come in great glory, they also ask that God would begin to inaugurate the final victory in the here and now, not only by forgiving sins, but also by healing people, thereby bringing glory to the divine name.

Later in the Lord's Prayer we ask the Father to "Deliver us from evil" (Mt 6:13), i.e., to free us from the power of Satan, the evil one. In other words we are asking God to free us from any evil, human or non-human that would try to separate us from God. It is arguable that some of the destructive tendencies we see at work in people's lives, e.g., a compulsive desire to self-harm, may be due, not just to severe depression, but also to the malign promptings of the enemy of our souls. The scriptures remind us, "For our struggle is not against flesh and blood, but against the rulers, against the authorities, against the powers of this dark world and against the spiritual forces of evil in the heavenly realms" (Eph 6:12). So in the prayer that follows the Our Father we go on to say, "deliver us from every evil and grant us peace in our day."

Having completed the Lord's Prayer we used to say: "Protect us from all anxiety." In his *Introduction to the Devout Life,* St Francis de Sales maintained that, "With the single exception of sin, anxiety is the greatest evil that can happen to a soul."[2] Interestingly, the word anxiety comes from the Latin meaning to "to press tightly, to narrow" and is related to the English words "anguish" and "angina." Psychologists have indicated, as we saw in earlier chapters, that many of our anxieties can be traced back to childhood, e.g., to a fear that we will lose the love, approval and acceptance of our carers. Because they are inclined to be mistrustful, anxious people are often self-absorbed. To a greater or lesser extent, they tend to be narrow minded and defensive where new ideas and relationships are concerned, including relationship with God. Fr. Ronald Rolheiser has suggested that when we pray "protect us from all anxiety" we really mean: "Protect us Lord, from going through life with a chip on our shoulders, angry at the world, full of paranoia, looking for someone to blame for our unhappiness."

Just before receiving holy communion we pray the following two prayers. Firstly we say, "Lamb of God you take away the sins of the world: grant us peace." *Shalom* was the Old Testament word for peace. It referred to anything that enjoyed integrity, completeness and well-being. *Erine* was the New Testament term for peace. It referred to "the tranquil possession of good things, happiness and above all health."[3] So when we pray for peace, we ask, not only for reconciliation with God and our neighbour, but also for wholeness of mind and body. Secondly, we go on to say in the words of the

---

2   Part IV, Chap 11.
3   Leon-Dufour, *Dictionary of the New Testament* (San Francisco: Harper & Row, 1980), 316.

Roman Centurion, "Only say the word and I shall be healed" (Mt 8:8). Many priests and lay people maintain that this petition refers to spiritual healing only. They are mistaken. The Lord wants to heal us as persons, in soul, mind and body. The Church indicates that this is, indeed, the case when it directs the celebrant to pray quietly, "Lord Jesus, with faith in your love and mercy I eat your body and drink your blood. Let it not bring me condemnation, but health in *mind* and *body.*"

A Testimony

Here is an example of what can happen. Many years ago I conducted a retreat for some lay people in London. On the final day we had a sharing session. Toward the end, Lucy, a middle aged woman, told us her remarkable story. Apparently she had entered a convent when she was eighteen. Then the night before her final profession she upped and left without telling anyone. Although she felt terribly guilty about her impulsive departure, she never returned. Sometime later she fell in love and married. Tragically, her first child died shortly after birth. Lucy believed - quite mistakenly of course - that God was punishing her for abandoning her religious vocation. She continued to believe this, in spite of the fact that her second child survived and enjoyed good health.

As the years passed her unresolved sense of guilt led to different kinds of neurotic problems. She developed severe agoraphobia. Because she was afraid of going outdoors she became a virtual prisoner in her own home, unable to visit friends, attend church, or to do her shopping. This went on for about fifteen years. Eventually Lucy was so anxious and depressed that she decided to take her own life. She saved up lots of pills with the intention of taking an overdose. Then one day in a state of despair and desperation she impulsively left her house and walked down the street in a daze. As she passed her parish church some primordial instinct drew her inside. Mass was in progress. Lucy knelt at the back. A silent scream of inner pain welled up inside her.

By now the priest had reached the consecration. As he extended his hands over the gifts he called on the Holy Spirit to descend upon them. At that very moment Lucy felt as if a bolt of lightning had hit her. A surge of energy passed through her body. She experienced a physical sense of heat and tingling. This went on for a few minutes. By the time it began to die down Lucy was a changed woman. Instead of feeling a sense of morbid guilt, she felt loved and cherished by an incredibly merciful God. Not only that, her depression had lifted, her agoraphobia had disappeared and she felt an inward sense of peace and joy. It was as if she had been born again. In fact she was so changed by this dramatic experience that for some time her husband found her hard to cope with. Instead of being dependant, as heretofore, she was now self-possessed and confident. He was able to say quite literally, "You are not the woman I married."

Conclusion

While it is good to visit shrines like Lourdes which are associated with healing, it is important to remember that the Eucharist can bring about healing of mind or body. As the host is placed on your tongue imagine the Lord is saying, "I love you, and because I love you I want what is best for you. My love is the answer to your deepest need. That love is upon you now and my Father is imparting his blessing of peace to you." When you say, Amen, it is an expression of confident trust in the benevolent, healing love of God.

I have seen many healings occur when the blessed sacrament is exposed. Sometimes, the celebrant will go down among the people blessing them as he passes with the monstrance. If people reach out with the fingers of faith, like the woman with the menstrual problem, they can experience healing of mind or body. I can recall a time when I was involved in a parish mission in a rural parish. As I walked down the aisle blessing people with the host, I got a subjective feeling as I passed by one of the benches that someone was being healed at that very moment. Two days later, when I was hearing confessions, a woman came into the confessional. At first, instead of speaking, she wept. Finally, when she pulled herself together emotionally she explained that she had suffered for many years from a very painful back complaint. Then she said that as I passed by with the monstrance, she experienced an inner faith conviction that she was being healed. The following day her back was completely pain free. When I asked her where she had been sitting, I found that it was exactly where I thought someone was being healed. Sometime later, as an act of thanksgiving to God, the same lady gave me a thousand pounds to give to charity. Soon afterwards, I was able to give five hundred to a travelling woman whose caravan had been deliberately set on fire, and another five hundred to a single woman, with two children, who was in danger of being evicted from her home because she was unable to pay an outstanding debt on her mortgage. We will return to the subject of Eucharistic healing in chapter twenty.

Preface for Mass of the Anointing of the Sick

"Father, all powerful and ever living God, we do well always and everywhere to give you thanks, for you have revealed to us in Christ the healer your unfailing power and steadfast compassion. In the splendour of his rising your Son conquered suffering and death and bequeathed to us his promise of a new and glorious world, where no bodily pain will afflict us and no anguish of spirit. Through your gift of the Spirit, you bless us, even now, with comfort and healing, strength and hope, forgiveness and peace. In this supreme sacrament of your love you give us the risen body of your Son: a pattern of what we shall become when he returns again at the end of time."

....

Chapter Twenty

Some Protocols for Healing Prayer

When one reads the New Testament it becomes apparent that, like Jesus, the apostles and disciples often prayed for people with the laying on of hands. Here are some examples. In Lk 4:40 we read that, "While the sun was setting, all those who had any who were sick with various diseases brought them to Him; and laying His hands on each one of them, he was healing them." Following the resurrection and ascension of Jesus the believers did much the same. In Acts 6:6 we are told that, "And these they brought before the apostles; and after praying, they laid their hands on them." Again in Acts 28:8 we are informed that, "it happened that the father of Publius was lying in bed afflicted with recurrent fever and dysentery; and Paul went in to see him and after he had prayed, he laid his hands on him and healed him." Finally in 1 Tim 4:14 St Paul said to his young protégé, " I remind you to kindle afresh the gift of God which is in you through the laying on of my hands."

Prayer Ministry in Today's Church

Prayer ministry with the laying on of hands is an aspect of a number of the sacraments such as Baptism, Confirmation, Ordination and Anointing of the Sick. In recent years it has also become a characteristic of the Charismatic Renewal Movement when praying for Baptism in the Spirit, healing, deliverance and the like. Pope Francis spoke about the practice in the context of person-to-person evangelisation when he said in par 128 of *The Joy of the Gospel*, If it seems prudent and if the circumstances are right, this fraternal and missionary encounter could end with a brief prayer [together with the laying on of hands] related to the concerns which the person may have expressed. In this way they will have an experience of being listened to and understood; they will know that their particular situation has been placed before God, and that God's word really speaks to their lives." In the words of the late John Wimber we can see all such opportunities for ministry with the laying on of hands as divine appointments[1] which are orchestrated by God and which can become power encounters.[2]

Some Guidelines

At this point we will look at some guidelines which help to express reverence for the person being prayed with, while being mindful of such issues as transference of a sexual nature, and the need to safeguard vulnerable children and adults.

1) It is very important that we only pray with a person when he or she has consented to having such prayer.

2) We should not presume to lay hands until the person being prayed with has said it is okay. The fact is, some people are not comfortable with bodily contact. We should be specific by asking, "do you mind if I/we place a hand/s on your head, or shoulder?"

3) It is better if a man prays with a man, and a woman with a woman. If there is more than one person ministering, it is better to have a man and a woman praying together, for either a man or woman. This helps to avoid the possibility of unconscious transference.[3]

---

1   "The Divine Appointment," in *Power Evangelism: Signs and Wonders Today* (London: Hodder & Stoughton, 1985), 61-73.

2   "The Power Encounter," in *Power Evangelism*, op. cit., 28-43.

3   Transference describes a situation where the feelings, desires, and expectations of one person are redirected and applied to another person. Most commonly, transference refers to a therapeutic setting, where a person in therapy may project certain feelings or emotions on the therapist. If a man prays for a woman, or *visa versa*, the unconscious imagery may be that of lovers, whereas if a man and woman pray for a person, male or female the unconscious imagery may be that of parents.

4) If you are laying hands on the person's head, e.g., when praying for baptism in the Spirit, or for healing, do so lightly without pressing down on the person.

5) If more than one person is ministering with the laying on of hands, it is helpful if there is an agreement about who is going to take the lead and do most of the talking. The other person/s quietly offer prayer support in English and/or tongues. If one of them gets a scripture, or a word from the Lord, they can share it when it seems appropriate.

6) Sometimes it can be good to check in with the person being prayed with to find out how he or she is feeling, or what they are aware of. This kind of feedback can be helpful because it can suggest what kind of ongoing prayer seems to be suitable. This would be particularly true when praying for inner healing, deliverance, or an in-filling of the Holy Spirit.

7) Pray with your eyes open. Look at the person you are praying with so you are aware of the nuances of his/her body language.

8) When they are being prayed with, some people may rest in the Spirit,[4] so it is important that a catcher be in position to ensure the person doesn't hurt him or herself.

9) Those involved in healing need to abide by a code of client confidentiality unless they have the client's permission to talk about a healing.

10) Until people can be inoculated with a vaccine against coronavirus, it is unlikely that the laying on of hands will be possible. In those circumstances clients, could be asked to put their own hands on the areas of their bodies that need healing.

---

4   Pat Collins, C.M., *Let the Spirit Lead* (Dublin: New Springtime Community, 2020), 166-172.

Some Spiritual Points to Keep in Mind

Many of these points have already been adverted to in the course of the book.

1] Because of justification by grace God is at work within us

When praying for a person, reject any exaggerated feelings of unworthiness by regarding them as a temptation from Satan, the accuser, the one who opposes the purposes of God. As a result of being justified by grace through firm faith in Christ's saving work on the cross we are qualified, through no merit of our own, to be channels of his blessing to others.

2] Minister in the Person of Jesus

When we are ministering to someone we believe that we are acting in the person of Jesus Christ (cf. Phil 2:13). While the Church teaches that bishops and priests act in the person of Jesus the head, e.g., to celebrate mass and forgive sins, all those who are baptised can minister in the person of Jesus. As was mentioned earlier in the book par. 521 of the *Catechism of the Catholic Church* assures us that, "Christ enables us to live in him all that he himself lived, and he lives it in us".

3] Be aware of the benevolence of God

Affirm the fact that God the Father is benevolent, all he has is ours (cf. Lk 15:31), if he has given us his Son, would he not give us all things in him? (Rm 8:32). The Father wants what is best for the person you are praying with.

4] Pray in the power of the Spirit

Affirm the fact that the Holy Spirit, the Lord and Giver of Life, is active in and through you. Focus on the reality that it is the same Spirit who raised Jesus from the powerlessness of death to glorious new life, who is at work in healing.

5]Praying within the will of God

Strive to pray for the person in accordance with the will of God, with the measure of faith you have received, trusting or expectant (cf. Rm 12:3). Sometimes expectant faith is possible either before or during the time of ministry because the Lord can give the praying person/s a word of knowledge.

Church Disciplinary Norms

In 2000 the Congregation for the Doctrine of the Faith issued an *Instruction on Prayers for Healing*. In a section entitled, "Disciplinary Norms" it included the following points.

1. It is licit for every member of the faithful to pray to God for healing. When this is organized in a church or other sacred place, it is appropriate that such prayers be led by an ordained minister.

2. Prayers for healing are considered to be liturgical if they are part of the liturgical books approved by the Church's competent authority; otherwise, they are non-liturgical.

3. Liturgical prayers for healing are celebrated according to the rite prescribed in the *Ordo benedictionis infirmorum of the Rituale Romanum* (28) and with the proper sacred vestments indicated therein.

4. It is absolutely forbidden to insert prayers of exorcism into the celebration of the Holy Mass, the sacraments, or the Liturgy of the Hours.

5. Those who direct healing services, whether liturgical or non-liturgical, are to strive to maintain a climate of peaceful devotion in the assembly and to exercise the necessary prudence if healings should take place among those present; when the celebration is over, any testimony can be collected with honesty and accuracy, and submitted to the proper ecclesiastical authority.

6. Authoritative intervention by the Diocesan Bishop is proper and necessary when abuses are verified in liturgical or

non-liturgical healing services, or when there is obvious scandal among the community of the faithful, or when there is a serious lack of observance of liturgical or disciplinary norms.

Since those disciplinary norms were published, the Church has become acutely aware of how important safeguarding measures are needed in order to protect children and vulnerable adults from any kind of abuse. As a result, all kinds of guidelines have been published both at a national and diocesan level. It is important that those who are involved in the healing ministry would not only be aware of the protocols recommended by the Church and the state, they need to conscientiously observe them.

Conclusion

Ministry in the power of the Spirit is an effective way of making the kingdom of God present in people's lives. There was a saying which was attributed to Hanina Ben Dosa, a contemporary of Jesus, "he whose actions exceed his wisdom, his wisdom shall endure, but he whose wisdom exceeds his actions, his wisdom shall not endure."[5] Not surprisingly, the apostles said similar things. For instance St Paul testified, "My message and my preaching were not with wise and persuasive words, but with a demonstration of the Spirit's power" (1 Cor 2:4)

It is important to remember that the ability to heal the sick is not nesessarily a sign of sanctity. Charisms are given to help others to grow in holiness but are not inevitably a sign that the person who exercises them is holy. As St thomas pointed out, a person in the state of mortal sin, could be used by God to heal others. So if healers want to boast because of the healings they have been instrumental in performing, they should boast in the Lord (1 Cor 1:31).

5   *Pirkei Avot- Ethics of the Fathers,* chapter 3, sec 12. https://www.myjewishlearning.com/article/pirkei-avot-ethics-of-the-fathers-4/

CHAPTER TWENTY ONE

HEALING SERVICES

For most Christians, the ministry of healing is a matter of person to person interaction. For example, it is not uncommon at the end of prayer meetings to see men and women praying with the laying on of hands for those who have asked for prayer, e.g., for healing. That said, some people who have a ministry of healing will try to cater for large numbers who want to be prayed with by organising healing services. In the past people like Kathryn Kulhman and Francis McNutt were well know for conducting large healing services. At the present time people like Randy Clark, Eddie Stone, Sr Briege McKenna and Damian Stayne run similar services.

I sometimes join Damian Stayne of the *Cor et Lemen Christi* community when he conducts, what he refers to as Catholic miracle rallies, in central London. They are attended by large crowds, and consist of prayer and praise, relevant teaching, and charismatic type healing ministry. Currently, Damian and his community rely heavily on words of knowledge to guide their prayer. What is striking is the fact that they get many such words before the services. I have heard members of his healing team share very precise and accurate information about who is going to be healed of what ailment and where exactly they are sitting. Straight away this raises the supernatural temperature. I have noticed that Damian will focus on the first one or two individuals who are mentioned. What is very striking is the fact that he expects them to experience healing right there on the spot. When it occurs, needless to say, it generates great excitement and heightened expectation in the hall. Not unexpectedly, that opens the door to many other healings. As various conditions are mentioned, members of Damian's community go to the designated people and pray with them. Anyone who is interested, can look at videos of healings at those services.[1]

The structure and content of a healing service

Over the years I have conducted many healing services for gatherings great and small. Like others, who are involved in the healing ministry, I have my own distinct way of organising such services. This outline is like a menu of dishes in a restaurant, or a colour pallet in an artist's studio which contains the kinds of elements that I often include in a service. That said, one or more of the elements, e.g., the sacramental anointing of the sick, testimony by a person who has been cured, or blessing with holy water can be omitted. Usually, the running order of a service can last anything between an hour and a quarter and two hours. It would go something like this.

1] Introduction by the leader who mentions briefly what is going to happen
People like to know what is going to happen so the leader explains that, for example, there will be
1. Opening hymn/s
2. Exposition of the Blessed Sacrament.
3. Liturgy of the word: a scripture reading and a homily
4. A testimony by a person who has experienced a healing
5. Sacrament of anointing
6. Brief prayer for one another in threes
7. Spontaneous prayer led by the leader
8. Blessing with the monstrance
9. After reservation of the host, blessing of water for the healing of the sick. Opportunity for those in attendance to bless themselves before leaving.

---

1   Google Damian Stayne.

2] Liturgy of the word

Following the opening hymn/s, exposition of the Eucharist and introduction, the liturgy of the word takes place.

- Reading, an appropriate text is proclaimed from either the Old or the New Testament
- Homily, which explains what the inspired author was saying while applying his words to the people at the service.
- Sometimes a person is invited to give a testimony, i.e., a brief account (5-10 mins) describing a healing he or she experienced in the past. It is a good way of evoking expectant faith in those who are present.

3] Liturgy of the anointing of the sick follows the liturgy of the word.

- Prayer over the people with arms outstretched
- Anointing of those with a serious ailment that needs regular attention of a doctor. I sometimes have them sit in the front seats in every second row so that I and other priests, who may be present, can have easy access to them all.
- Conclusion of the sacrament.

I always explain at healing services who it is that the Church stipulates are entitled to receive the anointing, i.e., baptized members of the Christian faithful who have reached the age of reason and who begin to be in danger due to sickness or old age. For example, the elderly who are weakened, even though no notable illness is present, may choose to participate in the ritual; those who face surgery due to serious illness; those who suffer serious mental illness. In other words, the health problem needs to be a serious and threatening one that requires the regular attention of a doctor. Although, I explain this, and ask those present not to come forward unless they satisfy the criteria, I have found that by and large they ignore my appeal and come forward in large numbers to be anointed, often for relatively trivial complaints. As a result, sad to say, I am less inclined to administer the sacrament of the anointing of the sick at healing services, firstly, because it takes an inordinate length of time to anoint the large numbers who come forward, and secondly, because they are not abiding by the Church's guidelines.

4] *Those attending the healing service break into groups of three to pray for one another.*

- Having spoken briefly about the fact that Christ has no hands on earth but ours, I encourage those present to pray briefly for one another possibly with the laying on of hands. The procedure is simple.
- Each person has an opportunity to say, if he or she wishes, what it is that they need prayer for.
- Then one person takes the lead, by saying the following short prayer or something like it, "Thank you Lord that your healing power is at work in my brother/sister, and that you are giving him/her your gift of peace in mind and body. Amen" The other person, silently or in tongues, backs up the spoken prayer.

5] *Spontaneous, Spirit guided prayer for the sick*

Like a number of others, I like to rely on words of knowledge to guide and empower me during healing services. I usually pray beforehand to ask Jesus to tell me who and what he wants to heal. When I get a spontaneous inspiration, I write it down to be used later during the service. Of course when the service is in progress I am open to receive a word of knowledge there and then. In this segment the order is usually as follows.

- One or two hymns, usually of praise in English and/or in tongues.
- Words of knowledge followed by spontaneous prayer for healing and/or deliverance
- If prayer teams are available, they go in twos to the people mentioned in order to pray briefly for them with the laying-on of hands.

6] Blessing with the monstrance throughout the church.

- Appropriate worship hymns are sung such as "Reach out and touch the Lord," "Be still and know that I am God" or "Father we adore you" as the priest goes down the central aisle blessing people on the left and right as he goes.

- When the priest returns to the sanctuary, he blesses the people. The congregation may sing, "O sacrament most holy," or "He is Lord." The host is returned to the tabernacle.

7] Blessing with holy water following reservation of the Blessed Sacrament

The people come forward to bless themselves by dipping their fingers in bowls of blessed holy water in front of the altar rails and then leave the church.[2]

Varying approaches and themes

Because I conduct so many healing services I like to vary them as much as possible by introducing new elements, varying the use of readings, the content of homilies and the like. Here are three examples of different approaches which have proved to be effective.

A] Touching the tallit

I have often read about the cure of the woman with the chronic bleeding problem in Mk 5:25-34, because it illustrates the importance of expectant faith in healing.[3] I discovered that one of the reasons the woman may have wanted to touch the hem of Jesus' garment was rooted in the fact that Mal 4:2 says, "the sun of righteousness will rise with healing in its rays." I have seen it suggested that this is a mistranslation, and that it could be more accurately translated to read, "the sun of righteousness will rise with healing in his tassels" i.e. the tassels of a tallit. Some scholars suggest that

---

2   The Vincentians, to whom I belong, have a Church approved prayer for the blessing of water to be used for healing purposes. See appendix three below.
3   See the homily on this text in chapter twenty two.

the Jews considered that, when the Messiah finally came, those who touched the tassels or hem on his tallit would be healed. That interpretation of Mal 4:2 would explain why we read in Mt 14:35-36, "And when the men of that place recognized Jesus, they sent word to all the surrounding country. People brought all their sick to him and begged him to let the sick *just touch the edge of his cloak*, and all who touched him were healed." It is my belief that this was probably the reason why the woman with the menstrual problem wanted to touch the hem of Jesus' cloak, "she thought, "If I just *touch his clothes*, I will be healed" (Mk 5:28).

When I was preparing for one healing service, the story of the healing of the woman with the menstrual problem came to mind. I was wondering whether there was some innovative way to highlight it in the service. Then I got an inspiration. I have a beautiful *tallit* which I sometimes wear when I'm praying. I wondered whether those who needed healing could touch it during the service if I wore it. Then the obvious thought occurred to me, "there is no point in wearing it myself, I'm not the Messiah." But then the idea came to me that I could lend it to Jesus, who truly is the Messiah, by placing the monstrance upon it and draping it out in front of the altar so that people could come forward and touch it. I can remember doing this when I conducted a healing service in Sicily a few years ago. I spoke about the expectant faith of the woman who touched the cloak of Jesus, and encouraged people needing healing to come forward and touch the *tallit* in the expectation that healing power could go out from Jesus to them, as it did to the woman in the Gospel. I was deeply moved as people came forward with such obvious devotion and reverence for the Eucharist, to touch the *tallit* with expectant faith. I noticed that many of them were in tears as they did so.

I was back in Sicily at the end of 2019 and met a woman who had attended that service. She told me that there were a number of reports of healing. She recounted one story which really impressed me. Apparently, a woman who had lost her husband a few years before had been suffering from depression and other ailments. Having touched the *tallit* with faith, all her depression lifted, and her other ailments were healed. When she returned home, she told her sister what had happened. The sister was so impressed that her faith grew to such a point that she too was healed of some medical problem that had been troubling her. Then that woman, in turn, told her daughter about her healing, and it had a similar knock on effect on her, with the result that a problem to do with childbearing was healed.

B] Cleansing the temple

A few years ago the late Myles Dempsey asked me to conduct a healing service at the New Dawn conference in Walsingham. Beforehand I asked God for inspiration. I was really surprised when it occurred to me that I should read the account in John's Gospel about the cleansing of the temple. At first it appeared to be irrelevant because it seemed to have nothing to do with healing. When I asked God to assist my understanding it suddenly occurred to me that the temple in Jerusalem could be seen as a symbol of the human body. After all, in 1 Cor 6:19, St Paul said, "Do you not know that your bodies are temples of the Holy Spirit."

As we know when Jesus visited the temple he was outraged by the fact that it was being profaned by the activities of those exchanging currency and selling animals for sacrifice. He was so indignant that, "he made a whip out of cords, and drove all from the temple area, both sheep and cattle; he scattered the coins of the money changers and overturned their tables" (Jn 2:15-16). I wondered if Jesus came to visit the temple of people's bodies, what would he find within them that would rouse his indignation. Surely it would be things like arthritis, heart disease, addiction, high blood pressure, thyroid problems and the like. They would evoke his righteous indignation as conditions that were an affront to the sanctity of the temple of the people's bodies. So I imagined that he would wield the whip of his ire while commanding them to leave the bodies of those present.

When we had the healing service, for well over one thousand people in a large tent, the gospel text about the cleansing of the temple was read. Then I gave a homily on its significance for us. Afterwards, in response to the Spirit's leading I mentioned many ailments. Having referred to each one in succession the people present loudly commanded the nominated affliction to leave the bodies of those present. Their passionate shouts resembled ardent prayers of deliverance. It turned out to be a very powerful experience which seemed to give expression to strong, expectant faith. Not surprisingly, in the aftermath of the service there were reports of a number of healings. For instance, a man wrote to me to say that he had been suffering from a very virulent form of cancer, which had unexpectedly gone into complete remission.

C] The Festal shout over strongholds
On another occasion when I was asked to conduct a healing service in Walsingham I asked God to help me to adopt a new approach and theme. What came to me in prayer was the story of the way the Jewish people captured the impregnable city of Jericho by means of a festal shout of victory. The outer wall of the city was six feet thick and about 20 to 26 feet high. The Israelites marched around the walls once every day for seven days with the priests and Ark of the Covenant. In Josh 6:5 we are told that the Lord said, "And when they make a long blast with the ram's horn, when you hear the sound of the trumpet, then all the people shall shout with a great shout, and the wall of the city will fall down flat." As Heb 11:30 says, "By faith the walls of Jericho fell, after the people had marched around them for seven days."

It struck me that we should read this text at the service and then give a homily which would suggest that our various sufferings and oppressions were like an impregnable stronghold which we are often unable to overcome by our own unaided efforts. But if like the Jewish people we marched round them shouting our praises and relying on the fact that, the battle was not ours but the Lord's, the strongholds of illness and oppression could be overcome and God's healing power released. During the service I encouraged the people to imagine that the stronghold of their pain and suffering was right there in the middle of the gathering. Having said this the people got up from their seats and began, quite spontaneously to march in a large circle around the tent shouting out their praises to God while declaring that the Holy Spirit, the Lord and giver of life, was tearing down those strongholds. That service not only led to healings but it also delivered people from spirits that had been oppressing them such as addictions, oppressions and obsessions which may have had a diabolical dimension.

Conclusion

Although, like others, I rely on words of knowledge to reveal God's will during healing services, I have a conviction that things like cancer and depression are rarely if ever in accord with God's will because they bare no fruit. It is significant that in Mk 11:12-25 Jesus cursed the fig tree for that very reason. Subsequently, it withered and died. It strikes me that, like Jesus, we have a right at healing services to curse cancer cells and to command them to cease to threaten the welfare of the body. Jesus is equally opposed to depression/anxiety. He wants us to forget about ourselves in out-going love of others, but in my experience deep depression/anxiety leads to self-absorption, and therefore, is not in accord with the will of God. So it seems to me that we are always authorised to pray a prayer of command at healing services against depression/anxiety, and to do so with expectant faith.

What I have said about conducting healing services is intended to be indicative rather than prescriptive. Each person who conducts one has to work out their own *modus vivendi*. However it is my hope that the foregoing points will prove to be a helpful resource. Healing services need to be well planned, while at the same time leaving room for surprises of the Spirit. I have found that if a music group is present and it plays appropriate songs, in a sensitive way, it can add greatly to the effectiveness of the service. I also know, only too well, how conducting healing services can be demanding and tiring. That said, quite often, by the grace of God, they become mystical times of blessing when heaven touches earth, and we have intimations of the coming of the new heavens and the new earth spoken about in Rev 21:1.

....

CHAPTER TWENTY TWO

HOMILY NOTES ON HOLISTIC HEALING

There is an outstanding passage in Mk 5:24-34 which describes the cure of the hemorrhaging woman. I often read it at healing services because, it not only highlights the importance of expectant faith, it also illustrates the holistic approach of Jesus to healing. Afterwards I preach a homily like the following.

It seems to me that the gospel reading we have just heard involves four interconnected elements.

A] Acknowledgment of Need

To begin with there is the acknowledgment of need. The haemorrhaging woman was one of the poor in spirit. She was not only suffering from a chronic menstrual problem, she also had to cope with its social and religious consequences. No wonder her condition is referred to as "a scourge" or "whip."

- Firstly, on a physical level her bleeding was a nuisance which caused anaemia and practical problems.

- Secondly, as far as the Jewish religion was concerned, she was ritually unclean (cf. Lev 15:19) and therefore excluded from the community and its worship, because it was thought that her uncleaness was communicable by touch. It also meant that she was unable to marry, and if she was already married she was unable to have sexual relations with her husband or to attend the synagogue.

- Thirdly, in Jewish thinking it was taken for granted that her affliction was a punishment for sin, so the woman had to cope with that religious stigma.

No wonder we are told that she had searched in vain for twelve years for a medical cure. She was painfully and even desperately aware of her urgent need for healing, and through it, for re-integration into the civil and religious community.

B] Hearing the Good News

Because faith comes by hearing the *rhema* word of Christ (cf. Rm 10:17) the woman needed to focus on the person and the words of Jesus. Presumably, she had not only heard about him, she had observed Jesus closely and listened to him speaking. His presence seems to have made a deep impression on her and his message seems to have found a place in her heart. Taken together they led to a rudimentary form of inspired knowledge. Jesus was the promised Messiah; a compassionate instrument of God's healing power.

C] Responding with expectant faith

As was mentioned already in chapter twenty one, Num 15:37-40 stated that Jewish men should wear a *tallit* with tassels. Later in Mal 3:20, there was a prophetic reference to the coming messiah which said, "the sun of righteousness will arise with healing in his tassels." At the time of Jesus, the people were familiar with the fact that the tassels of the messiah would have healing power. Presumably, that is why the woman with the bleeding problem had concluded that he was the Messiah and so she reached out to touch the tassels of Jesus' cloak. As someone who was ritually unclean, she did not want to make Jesus unclean by touching him, or even talking to him in public. Hers was a sensitive prayer of faith in action. Instead of saying, "If I touch even his clothes, I *may* be healed, *if* it is God's will," she said, "If I touch even his clothes, I *shall* be healed." Her inner sense of confidence was an example of what Jesus had in mind when he said, "I tell you, whatever you ask for in prayer, believe that you *have* received it and it will be yours" (Mk 11:24). The fact that her desire was in accordance with God's will, and that she had expectant faith, was confirmed by events. As soon as the woman, touched Jesus' garment, "*she knew in herself* that she was cured of her affliction" (Mk 5:29).

D] *Confession of faith*

When Jesus realised that power had gone out from him, he wanted to know who had touched him. At first sight, his question seemed a bit insensitive because it was calculated to draw attention to the woman and her embarrassing problem. But in fact, rather than being insensitive, Jesus was completing her healing. Knowing that she was the one, the woman spoke up. Her awareness of having been healed, was the reason she courageously overcame her feelings of timidity and revealed herself and what had happened to her to Jesus.

- Her public confession confirmed her physical healing,
- When she and Jesus acknowledged that fact it meant that she was no longer unclean and could, therefore, be fully reintegrated into the community.
- Furthermore, because she was no longer unclean, meant that her religious stigma had been removed.

So her healing was truly holistic, physical, social and religious. Jesus said to her, "Daughter, your faith has saved you. Go in peace and be healed of your scourge." The address, of 'daughter' is warm and confirms the woman's tri-fold healing. Jesus acknowledged that her unhesitating faith was the key to her recovery. Healings of the same kind can still be experienced today

Testimonies

A number of years ago, a woman confided in me by telling me that she had a problem similar to the woman in Mark's Gospel. Her periods were heavy and lasted most of the month. When she revealed her need in such a vulnerable way, I was deeply touched and had a desire to see her well. It struck me that her body was out of synchronization with the rhythms that govern the whole of nature such as the rising and setting of the sun, the ebb and flow of the tides, the passage of the four seasons, the waning and waxing of the moon etc. I felt that it was God's desire to re-establish a proper rhythm in her body. I got an inner conviction that God would heal her, not there and then, but at a time in the future which God would reveal to me.

So I told the woman this and often repeated that promise over a number of months. Then one day she came to see me. At one point during our conversation I had an inner sense that God's time had come to heal her. I urged her to stand and asked if it was all right to put a hand on her tummy as I prayed. Having received permission I prayed with expectant faith, believing that she was being granted the grace she needed. She did receive it. She was perfectly regular and normal from that day onwards.

Some time afterwards another woman told me about a similar problem. In her case, her periods were such that she would get so ill she would have to leave her work place and go home in a taxi in order to go to bed with the curtains shut. She might remain there for two days or more. When I prayed for her, she too was completely healed, as a result of having expectant faith.

Conclusion

There is a lot to be learned from the story of the healing of the woman with the bleeding problem. Firstly, one must move from a rather objective, intellectual acknowledgement of need to a more realistic, heartfelt awareness of one's inner poverty and vulnerability which expresses itself in an almost desperate desire for God's healing Spirit. In my experience, people often suppress that sense of need, for one reason or another, such as, fear of change, the possible loss of financial benefits, or perhaps forfeiting the sympathy of others. Secondly, instead of seeing God in the light of one's need, we should look at our need in the light of our trusting relationship with God and the alive and active word, which never returns to God empty without achieving its loving purpose. Thirdly, it is this kind of revelatory attention that increases our faith. As a result we may receive the grace that moves us from hesitant to expectant faith, the kind that opens us up to the healing power of God, as it did in the lives of the women with the menstrual problems.

CHAPTER TWENTY THREE

....

THE MYSTERY OF SUFFERING

When I was at school I can remember being deeply touched by a very poignant line from William Wordsworth's poem, *Lines Composed a Few Miles Above Tintern Abbey*. He described, "hearing oftentimes the still, sad music of humanity." How right he was. Although our world is beautiful in many ways, it is also a valley of tears, where there is a heartbreaking incidence of spiritual, emotional and physical suffering. While it is truly wonderful when people are healed in response to prayer, a question inevitably arises, why is it that God heals some people, while the pleas of many others seem to be ignored? Rabbi Harold Kushner, tried to answer that question from a Jewish point of view in his popular book, *When Bad Things Happen to Good People*.[1] I have heard disappointed and disillusioned people responding to the question about the whys and wherefores of suffering in all sorts of ways, such as, "because I'm forgotten . . . am cursed . . . am not worthy . . . am not loved by God . . . haven't sufficient faith . . . am being punished . . . perhaps there is no God there to respond, etc."

There is undoubtedly a tension in Christianity between the notion of redemptive suffering in the present and the prospect of partial and even complete healing in the future, especially when Christ comes again. In a document entitled, *Ethical and Religious Directives for Catholic Health Care Services*, the United States Conference of Catholic Bishops, reflected that tension when it wrote, "The mystery of Christ casts light on every facet of Catholic

....

1   (New York: Schocken Books, 1981).

health care... we see healing and compassion as a continuation of Christ's mission; to see suffering as a participation in the redemptive power of Christ's passion, death, and resurrection."[2] Scripture enables us to understand that tension between divergent truths from God's point of view. I want to refer to three texts in particular which have helped me greatly over the course of my lifetime.

Learning from the agony of Jesus in the garden

The first text is Mark's account of Jesus' agony in Gethsemane. On that occasion he prayed, "Abba, Father, everything is possible for you. Take this cup from me. Yet not what I will, but what you will" (Mk 14:36). In the first century the assertion that, "everything is possible for God" was not universally accepted in either the Greco-Roman or Jewish world. For example, the Stoics not only believed that God was apathetic and unmoved by human suffering, they also maintained that the world was governed by inexorable, impersonal, blind fate. For their part, the Jews were divided about the possibility of divine intervention. The Sadducees didn't believe that God could work miracles (cf. Acts 23:6-10). In our scientific, post-Enlightenment age many people do not believe that God can perform healings and miracles of a supernatural nature, in people's lives. However, Jesus asserted his conviction, on a number of occasions, that nothing was impossible to God. Time and time again, during his public ministry, he demonstrated the soundness of that belief when he performed healings, miracles and exorcisms. In Gethsemane it was no different. Jesus stated once again that he was convinced that nothing was impossible to his Father.

From a human point of view, the prospect of having to endure the mind numbing sufferings of passion week was almost too much for Jesus to contemplate. In a way this is surprising. Firstly, there was nothing unexpected about what faced him. On a number of occasions Jesus had spoken about his impending passion as an

2   Issued by USCCB, Nov, 2009, 6.

expression of the divine will. Secondly, in the wilderness Satan had tempted Jesus to abandon his vocation to be the suffering servant by relying on a miraculous intervention of God if he threw himself off the temple walls, in order to fulfil his mission in a painless way. Jesus had resisted that temptation. But in Gethsemane the same temptation seemed to be repeated. Although he was called to be the suffering servant, he seemed to ask his Father to change his plan. In other words, Jesus expressed his anguished hope that the Father might be able to usher in his kingdom without the necessity of redemptive suffering.[3] Having poured out his human feelings in an anguished way, Jesus did, however, remain submissive to God by saying, "Yet not what I will, but what you will." Although up to that point the Father had often revealed his will inwardly to Jesus, on this occasion there was no apparent communication. Instead, God was silent. His purposes were manifested in and through the unfolding events of the passion. Nevertheless our Lord courageously embraced God's saving plan. Afterwards, the author of Hebrews was to observe, "Although he was a son, he learned obedience from what he suffered" (Heb 5:8).

Whenever Christians have to endure suffering, they can share in the prayer of Jesus that the chalice of affliction would be removed, e.g., by means of a healing or miracle, but with Jesus they should also be prepared to say, "Yet not my will, but yours be done." Each year the Novena of Grace of St Francis Xavier is conducted in many churches. It is a time when members of the faithful present their different petitions, some of them requests for healing, to the Lord. When the novena prayer is recited, it contains the following words which echo the sentiments of Jesus in Gethsemane, "if what I ask is not for the glory of God or for the good of my soul, obtain for me what is most conducive to both." This prayer implies that while

3   Implicit in this temptation was an urge to switch from his vocation as the suffering servant to that of the military and political leader, of popular expectation, who would establish God's kingdom in a more painless way like king David of old.

healing in itself is a good thing and possible, God may not grant it because it might not be conducive to the purposes of divine providence or the greater good of one's soul.

St Zelie Martin, wife of St Louis Martin and the mother of St Therese of Lisieux had a lot of suffering to endure in the course of her life. For example, four of her children who were born before Therese, all died prematurely. When Therese was a young child, in 1876, Zelie was diagnosed as having breast cancer. Around that same time her sister, a Visitandine nun, died of tuberculosis. Zelie was well aware that her husband and daughters needed her, so she sought healing by going to Lourdes with three of her older children who, together with their mother, prayed fervently for a cure. In spite of being immersed several times in the water of the baths Zelie did not recover. As a very holy woman she was not lacking in faith. Nevertheless, soon after her return from the shrine, she died prematurely at the age of forty six in an attitude of courageous resignation to the will of God.

Power made perfect in weakness

There is a link to that last point in 2 Cor 12:7-9 where St Paul said, "there was given me a thorn in my flesh, a messenger of Satan, to torment me. Three times I pleaded with the Lord to take it away from me. But he said to me, "My grace is sufficient for you, for my power is made perfect in weakness." Although there has been a lot of speculation about the nature of the thorn that Paul had to endure, it could have been a health problem like epilepsy or eye trouble, if the truth be told, we have no idea what it was. Clearly, however, it weighed heavily on Paul and he wanted to be rid of it. But God refrained from responding to Paul's repeated entreaties to do that particular good, in order to do a greater good, namely that the apostle would remain humble in spite of the great revelations he had received. As a result, he would have little choice but to rely entirely on the grace of God in his weakness. As he testified in Phil 4:13, "I can do all things through him who strengthens me."

So when Jesus does not heal us, in spite of the fact that we asked him to do so, we have to believe in faith that there is a benevolent purpose implicit in such a refusal and that we can ask God to enlighten us as to what that purpose really is. St Paul himself, told us that one of the positive effects of suffering is that it schools the person in compassion. In 2 Cor 1:3-5 he said, "Blessed be the God and Father of our Lord Jesus Christ, the Father of mercies and God of all comfort, who comforts us in all our affliction, so that we may be able to comfort those who are in any affliction, with the comfort with which we ourselves are comforted by God." Perhaps the phrase, "wounded healer," has its origin in this realisation.

Redemptive suffering

When St John Paul II visited Knock Shrine in 1979, he spoke to the sick about the redemptive purpose of suffering. He said, "pain and sorrow are not endured alone or in vain. Although it remains difficult to understand suffering, Jesus has made it clear that its value is linked to his own suffering and death, to his own sacrifice. In other words, by your suffering you help Jesus in his work of salvation. This great truth is difficult to express accurately, but St Paul puts it this way, "in my flesh I complete what is lacking in Christ's afflictions for the sake of his body, that is, the Church" (Col 1:24). Your call to suffering requires strong faith and patience."[4]

St Therese Martin, like her mother, knew all about that truth. Soon after she entered the Carmelite convent in Lisieux, at the tender age of fifteen, her beloved father had several strokes and began to suffer from quite severe memory lapses, difficulty in speaking, fixations, unwarranted fears, periods of depression and exaltation, and a desire to run away and hide. Eventually he was sent to a mental hospital. Understandably, her father's illness caused Therese great distress. Sometime later, she herself was diagnosed as having tuberculosis. She suffered terribly, both physically and

---

4   *The Pope in Ireland: Addresses and Homilies* (Dublin: Veritas, 1979), 57.

emotionally. On one occasion she admitted, "Oh, if I didn't have the faith, I could never endure all this pain. I'm amazed that atheists don't commit suicide more often... Yes! What a mercy it is to have faith! If I didn't have faith, I should have killed myself without a moment's hesitation."[5] One of her sisters revealed that Therese begged prayers because, she said, the pain was enough to make her loose her reason. She asked that all poisonous substances be kept out of her reach, because in mind numbing pain, a person "no longer knowing what one is doing, one could easily take one's life."[6] In spite of her own prayers, and those of her family and community, Therese experienced little or no relief.[7]

As the time of her death approached, Therese said to her companions, "Don't be upset, dearest sisters, if I suffer a great deal and if you see no sign of happiness in me when I reach the point of death. Our Lord too died a victim of love, and see what his death agony of love was like!... Our Lord died on the cross in agony, yet this was the finest of deaths for love... The only example, indeed. Dying of love doesn't mean dying in transports of joy."[8] On the day she died, September 30th 1897, Therese suffered such violent temptations against faith that she was in total darkness. Several hours before her death, perspiration stood out on her forehead. She was agitated, close to despair and asked the sisters to sprinkle holy water on her. Her sister Pauline, i.e., Mother Agnes, was bewildered. She knew Therese was a saint, but her dying looked like that of a sinner. She went and prayed before a statue, saying, "Oh Sacred Heart of

5   Bernard Bro, *Little Way: The Spirituality of Thérèse of Lisieux* (New York: Alba House, 2014), 11.

6   Christopher O'Mahony, *St Therese of Lisieux: Her Last Conversations,* (Dublin: Veritas, 1975), 162-163.

7   Cf. Guy Gaucher, *The Passion of Therese of Lisieux* (New York: Crossroad, 1998).

8   *St. Thérèse of Lisieux: Her Last Conversations* (Washington: ICS Publications, 1977).

Jesus, I beg you, do not let my sister die in despair."[9] In a letter written to Leonie, shortly after their sister's death, Pauline described what had happened: "Our angel is in heaven. She gave up her last sigh at seven o'clock, pressing the crucifix to her heart and saying: "Oh I love You!" She had just lifted her eyes to heaven; what was she seeing!"[10]

Conclusion

Apparently the poet John Keats (1795-1821) was not a believing Christian. In a letter to his brother and sister in April of 1819 he presented what he viewed as a traditionally Christian, but as far as he was concerned, a mistaken conception of life as one of pure suffering from which we are to be "rescued" by a benevolent God. He said, "The common description of this world among the misguided and superstitious is 'a valley of tears' from which we are to be redeemed by a certain arbitrary interposition of God and taken to heaven." So it comes as no surprise to find that Keats rejected what he regarded as a fatalistic attitude as being too limited. He then went on to propose a new metaphor, of his own creation, that would more accurately sum up his understanding of the purpose of existence, "call the world if you please, the valley of soul-making." I have thought for a long time that there was a lot of truth in what Keats said. Suffering makes us either bitter or better. Although it is evil in itself, it can have many beneficial effects, when accepted with God's help, in a spirit of fortitude.

In Jer 17:9-10, we read, "The heart is deceitful above all things, and desperately sick; who can understand it? "I the Lord search the heart and test the mind." God often does this by means of the trials and tribulations of life, including sickness and disease. As Deut 8:2 says, "the Lord your God led you all the way in the desert these forty years, to humble you and to test you in order to know

9   Marie-Eugene, *Under the Torrent of His Love: Therese of Lisieux, a Spiritual Genius* (New York: Alba House, 1995), 56.
10   *St Therese of Lisieux: Her Last Conversations*, op. cit., 292.

what was in your heart." The desert for many people in today's society is the experience of ill-health of one kind or another. Carl Jung once observed, "There is no coming to consciousness without pain."[11] Suffering, therefore which is due to ill health, is an invitation not only to grow in self-awareness but also to grow in virtue. St Paul endorsed this point in Rom 5:3-5, "we also rejoice in our sufferings, because we know that suffering produces perseverance; perseverance, character; and character, hope. And hope does not disappoint us, because God has poured out his love into our hearts by the Holy Spirit, whom he has given us." So suffering which is accepted in a Christian way can lead to growth in holiness if not always in healing. It is a way of responding to the words of Jesus about the necessity of taking up one's cross daily and following him (cf. Mt 16:24).

11   *Contributions to Analytical Psychology* (Hong Kong: Hesperides Press, 2008), 193.

CHAPTER TWENTY FOUR

REFLECTIONS ON THE PANDEMIC

This book was written when I was cocooned during the coronavirus pandemic which began in early 2020. This worldwide phenomenon of sickness, which sadly has led to innumerable deaths, raises the question, why would God allow this to happen? To answer, we can begin by looking at something Jesus said in Mt 16:2-3, "When evening comes, you say, 'It will be fair weather, for the sky is red,' and in the morning, 'today it will be stormy, for the sky is red and overcast.' You know how to interpret the face of the sky, but you cannot interpret the signs of the times." They are significant events which, like so many dots, prophetic people can join together in such a way that they discern what on earth God is doing for heaven's sake. This notion was referred to during and after the Second Vatican Council. In par. 4 of the *Pastoral Constitution on the Church in the Modern World* we read, "the Church has always had the duty of scrutinizing the signs of the times and interpreting them in the light of the Gospel. Thus, in language intelligible to each generation, she can respond to the perennial questions which people ask about this present life and the life to come, and about the relationship of the one to the other."

Tribulations predicted

St John Paul II was one of those prophetic people who could interpret the signs of the times. In 1980, he said in par. 15 of *Dives et Misericordia* (Rich in Mercy), "If any of our contemporaries do not share the faith and hope which lead me, as a servant of Christ and steward of the mysteries of God, to implore God's mercy for humanity in this hour of history, let them at least try to understand the reason for my concern. It is dictated by love for man, for all that is human and which, according to the intuitions of many of our contemporaries, *is threatened by an immense danger* (my italics)."[1] A year later in 1981, St John Paul said to some pilgrims, "We must prepare ourselves, to suffer great trials before long, such as will demand of us a disposition to give up even life, and a total dedication to Christ and for Christ. With your and my prayer it is possible to mitigate this tribulation, but it is no longer possible to avert it, because only thus can the Church be effectively renewed."[2] Speaking about the coming time of tribulation Pope John Paul stated that it, "lies within the purposes of Divine providence. It is, therefore, in God's Plan, and it must be a trial which the Church must take up, and face courageously."[3]

At the beginning of 2020 we became aware of the coronavirus in China. Since then it has become a pandemic which has swept across the world with disastrous consequences. Not only has it resulted in many deaths, it has undermined the world's already vulnerable economic institutions which are floating on an ocean of debt. As Mervyn King, the former governor of the Bank of England, said in the introduction to his 2017 book *The End of Alchemy: Banking, the Global Economy and the Future of Money*,[4] "The crisis (of 2008) was not a failure of individual policy makers or bankers but of a system, and the ideas that underpinned it...There was a general misunderstanding of how the world economy worked." A little later he predicted, "Another crisis is certain, and the failure... to tackle the

---

1 When he announced the Extraordinary Jubilee of Mercy between Advent 2015 and Advent 2016, Pope Francis, quoted this point, with obvious approval of the notion that the world is threatened by an immense danger, in his papal bull *Misericordiae vultus*.

2 Pope John Paul II in Fulda, Germany (1980). http://archive.fatima.org/third-secret/fulda.as

3 Address given by Cardinal Karol Wojtyla during that 1976 Eucharistic Congress in Philadelphia. https://www.jkmi.com/apostolic-nuncio-calls-on-us-bishops

4 (New York: W. W. Norton & Company, 2017).

disequilibrium in the world economy makes it likely that it will come sooner rather than later." Coronavirus has already ignited this worldwide economic downturn. How long it will last, and what its effects will be, remains to be seen.

Jesus on the significance of tribulation

I would like to interpret current events in the light of something Jesus said about two disasters, one man made, the other natural.[5] They were referred to in Lk 13:1-5 where we read, "Now there were some present at that time who told Jesus about the Galileans whose blood Pilate had mixed with their sacrifices. Jesus answered, "Do you think that these Galileans were worse sinners than all the other Galileans because they suffered this way? I tell you, no! But unless you repent, you too will all perish. Or those eighteen who died when the tower in Siloam fell on them - do you think they were more guilty than all the others living in Jerusalem? I tell you, no! But unless you repent, you too will all perish."

Scripture scholars say that neither of the incidents which are mentioned by Luke in this passage was referred to in any other part of the bible or the secular histories of the time. Evidently, both of them took place during Jesus' lifetime within a stone's throw of one another in Jerusalem. We know very little about the Galileans who were murdered within the temple precincts. At Passover time, large crowds used to come to Jerusalem to offer sacrifice in the temple. It is quite possible that during a disturbance that occurred there, Pilate's troops quelled the unrest in a violent way that led to loss of life. Evidently, the blood of those who were wounded and killed was mixed, in a sacrilegious way, with that of their animal sacrifices. Josephus, the Jewish historian, recalled a similar incident in his *Antiquities*, when a number of Samaritans were executed on Pilate's orders following a religious protest.

---

5   Whereas coronavirus is a natural disaster, the economic downturn is a man-made catastrophe.

As far as the collapse of the tower which killed eighteen men, is concerned, we know a little more about it. Archaeologists, are fairly sure that they have discovered its ruins near the spring of Siloam (cf. Jn 9:7), some distance south of Herod's fortress. We know that Pilate had been trying to improve the water supply to the city and was embezzling temple revenues to finance the project. The Pharisees argued that the labourers who worked on the building of the aqueduct were wrong to do so. The collapse of the tower may have been due to the fact that its foundations had been undermined by the construction work nearby.

In the Jewish theology of Jesus' time, the people would have assumed that the victims in both incidents had lost their lives as a divine punishment for their grievous sins. As Eliphaz said to Job: "Consider now: who, being innocent, has ever perished? Where were the upright ever destroyed?" (Job 4:7). The same belief was evident in the story of Jesus' cure of the blind man, "His disciples asked him, "Rabbi, who sinned, this man or his parents, that he was born blind?" (Jn 9:2). Jesus surprised the enquirers when he said that the man's blindness had nothing directly to do with his own sins or those of his parents.

As far as Jesus was concerned although the people who died were sinners, they were no more so than anyone else. As Joachim Jeremias pointed out in his *New Testament Theology*, "In Lk 13:1-5, Jesus expressly attacks the dogma that misfortune is a punishment for the definite sins of particular people. Rather, suffering is a call to repentance, a call which goes out to all. Whereas his contemporaries ask, 'Why does God send suffering?' the disciples of Jesus are to ask, '*For what* does God send suffering?' Jeremias goes on to say, "One answer would be, God allows suffering, in order to summon people to repentance lest they suffer a greater catastrophe."[6]

The reply of Jesus does not support the mistaken notion that an angry God inflicts suffering and death upon sinners as a

6   (London: SCM Press, 1971), 183. Reference to "a greater catastrophe" has the general judgement rather than the great tribulation in mind.

punishment. Like people who suffer from lung disease as a result of smoking, sinful people are the authors of their own misfortunes. Understood in that way their sufferings can be seen as self-inflicted rather than God-inflicted. But if the truth be told, God, who is unconditionally loving, hates sin but loves the sinners and does not want them to suffer. Secondly, given the fact that people do suffer affliction, it can be seen as a happy fault in so far as God can bring good from evil. For example, when Joseph met his brothers who had sold him into slavery in Egypt, he said to them, "You intended to harm me, but God intended it for good to accomplish what is now being done, the saving of many lives" (Gen 50:20). God has allowed, but not wanted, the current pandemic. In words taken from the *Exultet* of Easter Sunday the pandemic is paradoxically, a "happy fault." The coronavirus infection contains an implicit invitation to come to one's senses, like the prodigal son, and to return to God the merciful Father. That notion seems to be implicit in Hos 6:1-2 which says, "Come, let us return to the Lord; for he has torn us, that he may heal us; he has struck us down, and he will bind us up. After two days he will revive us; on the third day he will raise us up, that we may live before him."

Coronavirus a call to conversion

Postmodernism maintains that the human mind cannot know absolute truth, so at best all truth is probable, partial, and provisional. Writing in par. 91 of his encyclical *Faith and Reason*, St John Paul II observed, "the time of certainties is irrevocably past, and the human being must now learn to live in a horizon of total absence of meaning, where everything is provisional and ephemeral. In their destructive critiques of every certitude, several authors have failed to make crucial distinctions and have called into question the certitudes of faith."

It is not surprising therefore that in our secular society many citizens fail to acknowledge God's ultimate authority in the realm of morality. In this regard one is reminded of what Judges 21:25

says, "In those days there was no king in Israel [no ultimate author-
ity]. Everyone did what was right in his own eyes." Aldous Huxley,
acted as spokesman for those who, in our post-truth society,
espouse ethical relativism when he wrote in the mid twentieth century, "I had motives for not wanting the world to have a meaning;
and consequently assumed that it had none, and was able without
any difficulty to find satisfying reasons for this assumption. The
philosopher who finds no meaning in the world is not concerned
exclusively with a problem in pure metaphysics. He is also concerned to prove that there is no valid reason why he personally
should not do as he wants to do. For myself, as no doubt for most
of my friends, the philosophy of meaninglessness was essentially
an instrument of liberation from a certain system of morality. We
objected to the morality because it interfered with our sexual freedom. The supporters of this system claimed that it embodied the
meaning - the Christian meaning, they insisted - of the world.
There was one admirably simple method of confuting these people
and justifying ourselves in our erotic revolt: we would deny that the
world had any meaning whatever."[7] It strikes me that this relativist
mentality is implicit in the worldview of those who argue for the
legitimacy of such things as sex outside marriage, same sex marriage, abortion, and euthanasia.

In my opinion, we have to understand the tribulations we are
currently enduring within this wider moral and religious context.
Paradoxically, from a theological point of view, it could be said that
current tribulations are at once a painful consequence of modern
society's wilful forgetfulness of God, and a mercy in so far as God
allows us to be disciplined by painful events, such as the current
pandemic, as a way of calling those who are contrite to repentance.
It is as if Jesus is saying to the people of our time, "Satan demanded
to have you, that he might sift you like wheat" (Lk 22:31). The
Lord has allowed Satan to do so for a good purpose, by means of

7   Aldous Huxley, *Ends and Means: An Inquiry into the Nature of Ideals* (London:
     Chatto & Windus. 1946), 273.

the painful health and economic crises we are currently enduring. As Heb 12:11 says, "No discipline seems pleasant at the time, but painful. Later on, however, it produces a harvest of righteousness and peace *for those who have been trained by it.*" It is my guess that the current tribulation will be met by mixed reactions, as was the bubonic plague in the fourteenth century.[8]

1) Some people will turn away from God in an angry resentful way believing that there is no deity, or that God is heartless and has ignored them in their time of need. As a result, they may be inclined to eat drink and be merry, believing in a rather despairing way that they are, "without hope and without God in the world" (Eph 2:12).

2) Others will be like the Egyptians of old who as Wisdom 17:12-13; 15 tells us were overwhelmed by irrational fears, "Fear is nothing but the failure to use the help that reason gives. When you lack the confidence to rely on reason, you give in to the fears caused by ignorance... as they surrendered themselves to the sudden, unexpected fear that came over them." No wonder the poet W. H. Auden referred to the contemporary era as "the Age of Anxiety."[9]

3) Some people will mistakenly interpret the coronavirus as the beginning of the apocalypse, the end times spoken about in scripture. While it is an intimation of the great tribulation, that time has not yet come.[10]

4) Others, however, may be like the prodigal son who, humbled by his tribulations, came to his senses and decided to return to his father and his Jewish origins, values and beliefs. Like him, many modern men and women may

---

8   Cf., Philip Ziegler, *The Black Death* (London: Penguin, 1976).

9   W. H. Auden, *The Age of Anxiety: A Baroque Eclogue* (Princeton: Princeton University Press, 2011).

10 For a discussion of the prophetic signs that will precede the Second Coming of Jesus see my, *Countdown to Doomsday: How Our World will End.* (Luton: New Life, 2020).

respond consciously or unconsciously to the words, "Seek the Lord while he may be found, call upon him while he is near: Let the wicked forsake his way, and the unrighteous man his thoughts: and let him return to the Lord, and he will have mercy upon him; and to our God, for he will abundantly pardon" (Is 55:6-7).

5) I'm sure there will be a minority of believers, who will be so trusting in God, that no matter what happens, they will praise God in an unconditional way as they anticipate the blessings to come. In Hab 3:17-19, there are verses which express their hope filled attitude, "Though the fig tree should not blossom, nor fruit be on the vines, the produce of the olive fail and the fields yield no food, the flock be cut off from the fold and there be no herd in the stalls, yet I will rejoice in the Lord; I will take joy in the God of my salvation. God, the Lord, is my strength; he makes my feet like the deer's; he makes me tread on high places."

Conclusion

If people fail to hear and respond to God's voice in and through current events, I suspect that, even though those trying events will eventually come to an end, they will only be succeeded by even greater tribulations in the future. God will continue to knock on the door of the hearts of those who are no longer mindful of the divine presence or purposes, in the hope that they will finally undergo a change of mind which will lead them to accept that the truth is not a proposition but rather a person the person of Jesus (cf. Jn 14:6) and that we should avoid doing what is evil in God's eyes (cf. Ps 51:4).

The question is, will people have to experience an even more devastating tribulation, before they realise that the current pandemic and its economic aftermath is a dress rehearsal for the advent of the Antichrist and the great tribulation (cf. Rev 7:14) which will precede the second coming of Jesus. If we are anxious about what is happening in the world, at the present time, we should be even more preoccupied by the second coming of Jesus when all the living and the dead will have to stand before the judgement seat of God. Those who are in the state of grace will enter eternal glory and those who are not, will depart to a state of eternal alienation from God, their true selves and from others. That will be the greatest catastrophe of all, one which we all need to guard against.

In the meantime as long as the current pandemic continues, individuals and groups of believers can pray, not only for the conversion of sinners, but they can also witness to the divine mercy by praying with faith for the healing of people who are afflicted by coronavirus.

PRAYER FOR IRELAND

Lord we thank you for the countless blessings you have poured out on our country in the past. We praise you for the way in which your grace found expression in many generous and loving lives. We are grateful for the prosperity we have enjoyed. However, we regret, that the flame of the Spirit has sometimes been quenched by an idolatrous pursuit of power, pleasure, popularity and possessions. We confess Lord, that many of us have gone astray, and selfishly rewritten the commandments to suit ourselves. We believe that you came to cast fire on the earth and we long for you to renew your wonders in our day as by a new Pentecost. Help us to fan the embers of our smouldering faith into a lively flame, especially by means of regular periods of scripture reading, personal and family prayer, together with acts of self-denial. Mary mother of Jesus, we entrust Ireland to your motherly care. In the past our people remained faithful to your Son in times of persecution. We pray now that we may also remain faithful in times of tribulation. Amen.

Chapter Twenty Five

Consecration of One's Hands for Healing Ministry

Believing as I do that there is no growth or blessing in the Christian life without preceding desire I have asked myself many times, "what grace do you most desire at this particular time in your life?" At one point I found myself replying, I want to have a deeper faith conviction about the love Jesus has for me in order that I might love others better than I do at present. I prayed for that grace for many months without any apparent response. Then I went on my annual retreat with some of my fellow priests. Each evening we spent an hour of adoration in the presence of the Eucharist exposed in the monstrance.

On one of the evenings I was sitting in my seat contemplating the host. Suddenly in my mind's eye I saw Jesus standing in front of the altar. He wasn't at all like what I expected. He was young and attractive looking. He had short hair and no beard or moustache. He wore a simple off white, one-piece garment and red light was streaming from his right palm and white light from his left palm. At first, his hands were held in a downward position slightly away from his body. Then he slowly raised his palms. There was a momentary flash of light from each. The flashes reminded me of the burst of light that comes from a lighthouse on the sea coast. Then Jesus lowered his extended hands in front of him, in an attitude of blessing, and I found myself sitting in the gentle glow of the converging beams of red and white light. Inwardly I knew that I was sitting in the light of God's mercy and love. My spirit seemed to be illumined. I was immediately reminded of the words, "We have known and believe the love God has for us" (1 Jn 4:16). It encapsulated my new-found awareness which filled me with peace.

When I reflected in a prayerful way on that experience I could see that the Lord had answered my prayer in a wonderful manner. I was also reminded of a verse in Hab 3:4 which says, "Rays came forth from his hands where his power lies hidden." It struck me that the Lord was urging me to pray with people as an expression of his divine love. We have already adverted to the fact, in chapter twenty, that the laying on of hands was a feature of New Testament ministry. Ever since then, when I'm praying with people, I believe that the invisible light of God's merciful love is flowing through my hands. Indeed, there have been times when I have sensed heat in my palms and a sensation like pins and needles in my arms. I believe that it is caused by the same Holy Spirit that flowed through Jesus. I have found that prayers like these can be powerful and effective.

In more recent years I read these illuminating words in par 344 of the *Diary* of St Faustina. They enabled me to have a deeper understanding of the meaning and implications of the vision I have just described.

"One evening as I entered my cell, I saw the Lord Jesus exposed in the monstrance under the open sky, as it seemed. At the feet of Jesus I saw my confessor, and behind him a great number of the highest ranking ecclesiastics, clothed in vestments the like of which I had never seen except in this vision; and behind them, groups of religious from various orders; and further still I saw enormous crowds of people, which extended far beyond my vision. I saw the two rays coming out from the host, as in the Divine Mercy image, closely united but not intermingled; and they passed through the hands of my confessor, and then through the hands of the clergy and from their hands to the people, and then they returned to the host... And at that moment I saw myself once again in the cell which I had just entered."

The words of St Faustina helped me to understand that Christ in the Eucharist pours forth the invisible light of his mercy and love, which enters the hands of the clergy who have the task of mediating that merciful love to the laity by means of the sacraments, e.g., reconciliation, the Eucharist and the anointing of the sick. They can also mediate the love of God by means of the laying on of hands in prayer ministry. The laity too, who share in the priesthood of Christ, can pray for one another in much the same way. Hopefully those who have experienced the love of God in the form of holistic healing will later go on to reflect that love back to Jesus in the Blessed Sacrament by means of praise, thanksgiving and adoration.

Prayer to consecrate one's hands for healing

You will remember that St Teresa of Avila said that nowadays Jesus has no hands on earth except yours and mine. He wants to use them, as he used his own, in order to minister healing to the suffering people of our day, many of whom are "harassed and helpless, like sheep without a shepherd" (Mt 9:36). Knowing this, I often consecrate my hands to God's healing purposes. Why not stretch out your hands right now as an offering to the Lord while saying the following prayer.

> "Lord Jesus, in the modern world you have no hands but mine. Today, I solemnly offer you my hands. May the light of your merciful love shine forth from the Eucharistic host into them, so that I in my turn may use them to bring the light of your merciful love to others as I lay my hands on them in order to pray for graces such as deliverance, healing and blessing. I thank you that you are accepting my offering, that your are consecrating my hands to your service, so that they may be instruments of your saving and loving purposes in the world of today. Amen."

....

SPIRITUAL WARFARE PRAYER

Heavenly Father, I love you, I praise you, and I worship you. I thank you for sending Your Son Jesus who won the victory over sin and death for my salvation. I thank you for sending your Holy Spirit who empowers me, guides me, and leads me into fullness of life. I thank you for Mary, my heavenly mother, who intercedes with the Holy Angels and saints for me.

Lord Jesus Christ, I place myself at the foot of your cross and ask you to cover me with your precious blood which pours forth from your most Sacred Heart and your most holy wounds. Cleanse me, my Jesus, in the living water that flows from your heart. I ask you to surround me, Lord Jesus, with your holy light.

Heavenly Father, let the healing waters of my baptism now flow back through the maternal and paternal generations to purify my family line of Satan and sin. I come before you, Father, and ask forgiveness for myself, my relatives, and my ancestors, for any calling upon powers that set themselves up in opposition to you or that do not offer true honour to Jesus Christ. In Jesus' holy name, I now reclaim any territory that was handed over to Satan and place it under the Lordship of Jesus Christ.

By the power of your Holy Spirit, reveal to me, Father, any people I need to forgive and any areas of un-confessed sin. Reveal aspects of my life that are not pleasing to you Father, ways that have given or could give Satan a foothold in my life. Father, I give to you any un-forgiveness; I give to you my sins; and, I give to you all ways that Satan has a hold of my life. Thank you, for your forgiveness and your liberating love.

Lord Jesus, in your holy name, I bind all evil spirits of the air, water, ground, underground, and netherworld. I further bind, in Jesus' Name, any and all emissaries of the Satanic headquarters and claim the precious blood of Jesus on the air, atmosphere, water, ground and their fruits around us, the underground and the netherworld below.

Heavenly Father, allow your Son Jesus to come now with the Holy Spirit, the Blessed Virgin Mary, the holy angels and the saints to protect me from all harm and to keep all evil spirits from taking revenge on me in any way. *(Repeat the following sentence three times: once in honour of the Father, once in honour of the Son, and once in honour of the Holy Spirit).* In the Holy Name of Jesus, I seal myself, my relatives, this room *(place, home, church, car, plane, etc...)*, and all sources of supply in the precious blood of Jesus Christ.

(To break and dissolve all Satanic seals, repeat the following paragraph three times in honour of the Holy Trinity because satanic seals are placed three times to blaspheme the Holy Trinity.) In the holy name of Jesus, I break and dissolve any and all curses, hexes, spells, snares, traps, lies, obstacles, deceptions, diversions, spiritual influences, evil wishes, evil desires, hereditary seals, known and unknown, and every dysfunction and disease from any source including my mistakes and sins. In Jesus' name, I sever the transmission of any and all Satanic vows, pacts, spiritual bonds, soul ties, and satanic works. In Jesus' name, I break and dissolve any and all links and effects of links with: astrologers; channelers; clairvoyants; crystal healers; crystals; fortune tellers; mediums; the New Age Movement; occult seers; palm, tea leaf, or tarot card readers; psychics; satanic cults; spirit guides; witches; witch doctors; and, voodoo. In Jesus' name, I dissolve all effects of participation in séances and divination, Ouija boards, horoscopes, occult games of all sorts, and any form of worship that does not offer true honour to Jesus Christ.

Holy Spirit, please reveal to me through a word of knowledge any evil spirits that have attached themselves to me in any way. *(Pause and wait for words to come to you, such as: anger, arrogance, bitterness, brutality, confusion, cruelty, deception, envy, fear, hatred, insecurity, jealousy, pride, resentment, or terror. Pray the following for each of the spirits revealed.)* In the name of Jesus, I rebuke you spirit of _____. I command you to go directly to Jesus, without manifestation and without harm to me or anyone, so that he can dispose of you according to his holy will.

I thank you, Heavenly Father for your love. I thank you, Holy Spirit for empowering me to be aggressive against Satan and evil spirits. I thank you, Jesus, for setting me free. I thank you, Mary, for interceding for me with the holy angels and the saints.

Lord Jesus, fill me with charity, compassion, faith, gentleness, hope, humility, joy, kindness, light, love, mercy, modesty, patience, peace, purity, security, tranquillity, trust, truth, understanding, and wisdom. Help me to walk in your light and truth, illuminated by the Holy Spirit so that together we may praise, honour, and glorify our Father in time and in eternity. For you, Lord Jesus, are, "the way, the truth, and the life" (Jn 14:6), and you "…have come that we might have life and have it more abundantly" (Jn 10:10). "God indeed is my Saviour; I am confident and unafraid. My strength and courage is the Lord, and he has been my Saviour" (Is 12:2).[1] Amen."

---

1   Fr Robert de Grandis, SSJ. https://prayersroom.com/fr-robert-de-grandis-ssj-spiritual-warfare-prayer/

....

FORGIVENESS PRAYER

Lord Jesus Christ, I ask for the grace today to forgive everyone in my life. I know that you will give me strength to forgive. I let go of all resentment toward you because of hardships, death and sickness in the family. I surrender to you today in faith and trust; you love me more than I love myself, and want my happiness more than I desire it for myself. Jesus, you are Lord of my life. Please come into my heart in a deeper way and remove anything that would block the flow of your love. Please give me the grace to rest in your arms and allow myself to be loved by you.

Lord, because you have forgiven me, I can forgive myself for sins, faults, and failings. For all that is truly bad in myself or all that I think is bad, I truly forgive myself. For any delving into the occult, Ouija boards, horoscopes, séances, fortune telling or using lucky charms; for any calling upon sources of power apart from you; for taking your name in vain; for not worshipping you; for hurting my parents; for getting drunk or using drugs; for sins against my purity; for adultery; for abortion; for stealing or lying; I truly forgive myself today. I let go of all self-directed negativity. I release the things held against myself and make peace with myself today.

I now stand before you as an intercessor and extend forgiveness to my ancestors for acts of negativity and unloving behaviour and attitudes. I come before you, Lord, on behalf of everyone in my family tree and apologize for any sinful actions. Let forgiveness flow through my family tree. Let the wounds of the past be healed through my act of forgiveness today. Thank you, Lord.

I forgive my mother, Lord. I forgive her for times she may have hurt me, resented me or punished me unfairly. I forgive her for preferring my brothers and sisters; I forgive her for telling me I was dumb, ugly, stupid, the worst of the children, or that I cost the family a lot of money. I forgive her for rejecting me, abandoning me, or attempting to abort me. I forgive her for telling me I was unwanted, an accident or a mistake. I forgive her for any lack of hugs and kisses. For any ways she did not provide a deep satisfying mother's blessing I truly forgive her today. I pray for her today, and ask God's blessing upon her.

I forgive my father, Lord. I forgive him for any non-support, lack of companionship, drinking, severe punishments, emotional abuse, desertion or unfaithfulness to my mother. I forgive him for not showing his love; lack of hugs and kisses, tenderness and intimacy. For any ways that I did not receive a deep, satisfying father's blessing I do forgive him today. I pray for him, and ask God's blessing upon him.

I forgive my sisters and brothers for any unloving acts and negativity. I forgive those who rejected me, lied about me, resented me, physically harmed me, or competed for my parent's love. I forgive all blood-relatives for harm done to our family. I forgive all in-laws for any abuses and expressions of negativity and lack of love. I pray for them and ask God's blessing upon them.

I forgive my spouse for any lack of love, lack of affection, lack of consideration, lack of support, or lack of communication; I forgive my spouse for faults, failings and weaknesses. I ask God's blessing on my spouse today.

I forgive my children today. I forgive them for lack of respect, lack of obedience, lack of love, lack of attention, and lack of understanding. I forgive them for their bad habits, for falling away from the Church, and for any action that disturbed me. I pray for them and ask God's blessing upon them.

I forgive my friends. I forgive them for letting me down, gossiping about me, borrowing money and not returning it, and encouraging sinful behaviour. I pray for them and ask God's blessing upon them.

I forgive my neighbours. For any act of negativity, for lack of consideration, for prejudice, for running down the neighbourhood, I do forgive them today. I pray for them and ask God's blessing upon them.

I forgive priests, nuns, brothers and bishops, and the Pope for lack of support, lack of friendliness, pettiness, bad sermons, for any hurt they may have inflicted. I pray for them and ask God's blessing upon them.

I forgive my employer. I forgive him/her for not paying me enough money, for not appreciating my work, for being unkind and unreasonable, for being angry or unfriendly, for not promoting me, for not complimenting me on my work. I pray for my employer today and ask God's blessing upon him/her.

I forgive all professional people. I forgive lawyers, barristers and solicitors for any harm they may have done. I forgive school teachers for humiliating me and imposing unfair punishments; for lack of warmth; for not encouraging my potential.

I forgive doctors, nurses, and other medical professionals for treating me unjustly. I pray for them and ask God's blessing upon them.

I forgive people in public service. I forgive those who have passed laws opposing Christian values. I forgive police for any abuses. I pray for them today and ask God's blessing upon them. Heavenly Father, I now forgive every member of society who has hurt me in any way.

I forgive those who have rejected me or hurt me by criminal action, sexual aggression or obscene actions. I forgive the strangers and nameless perpetrators of evil in society. I forgive those who have defrauded me or defamed my character. I forgive those to whom I cannot go directly and face with my anger: the burglar who got away, the rapist, the murderer, unknown carriers of disease, wartime aggressors. I pray for them today and ask God's blessing upon them.

Heavenly Father, I now forgive by an act of my will the one person in life who has hurt me the most. The one who is hardest to forgive, I now choose to forgive. I also make peace with the one family member, the one friend, and the one member of the clergy who has hurt me the most in life. I pray for them today and ask God's blessing upon them. Thank you Heavenly Father for setting me free. In Jesus holy name Amen.

If you now feel better, then you have just experienced healing through forgiveness. You should feel lighter and much more peaceful. Forgiveness is an act of the will, not the emotions. As you choose to forgive, God will empower that choice and bring it, in time, from your head to your heart. It is recommended that you pray this prayer daily, perhaps for nine days as a novena. Ask the Holy Spirit to open your heart to deeper levels of forgiveness. This will heighten your awareness of the need to forgive and increase your "forgiveness consciousness."[1]

---

1   Robert DeGrandis S.S.J. and Betty Tapscott, *Forgiveness & Inner Healing* (Hartselle: Betty Tapscott, 2007).

Appendix Three

....

Blessing of the oil of gladness taken from the Roman Ritual

(Use regular, 100% pure oil. The priest vests in surplice and purple stole)

P. Our help is in the name of the Lord.

R. Who made heaven and earth.

P: O oil, creature of God, I exorcise you by God the Father (+) almighty, who made heaven and earth and sea, and all that they contain. Let the adversary's power, the devil's legions, and all of Satan's attacks and plots be dispelled and driven far from this creature, oil. Let it bring health in body and mind to all who use it, in the name of God (+) the Father almighty, and of our Lord Jesus (+) Christ, His Son, and of the Holy (+) Spirit, as well as in the love of the same Jesus Christ our Lord, who is coming to judge both the living and the dead and the world by fire.

R. Amen.

P: O Lord hear my prayer.

R: And let my cry come to you.

P: May the Lord be with you.

R: And with your spirit.

P: Let us pray. Lord God almighty, before whom the hosts of angels stand in awe, and whose heavenly service we acknowledge; may it please you to regard favourably and to bless (+) and sanctify (+) this creature, oil, which by your power has been pressed from the juice of olives. You have intended it for anointing the sick, so that, when they are made well, they may give thanks to you, the living and true God. Grant we pray, that those who will use this oil, which we are blessing (+) in your name, may be protected from every attack of the unclean spirit, and delivered from all suffering, all infirmity, and all wiles of the enemy. Let it be a means of averting any kind of adversity from man, redeemed by the precious blood of your Son, so that he may never again suffer the sting of the ancient serpent. Through Christ our Lord.

R. Amen

Blessing of Water in Honour of St Vincent de Paul

(Formerly reserved to the Congregation of the Missions and approved by the Congregation of Sacred Rites, March 16th 1882)

Let us pray.

Holy Lord, almighty Father, everlasting God, who, in pouring out the grace of your blessing on the bodies of the sick, surround your creatures with your generous love; listen as we call on your holy name, and by the prayers of Blessed Vincent, your confessor, free your servants from illness and restore them to health, and then hasten their convalescence by your sure hand, strengthen them by your might, shield them by your power, and give them back in full vigour to your holy Church; through Christ our Lord.

All: Amen.

Then a medal or a relic of St. Vincent de Paul is immersed in the water, and it is held there until the following prayer is concluded:

Lord, bless + this water, so that it may be a saving remedy for men and women; and grant that, by the prayers of Saint Vincent, your confessor, whose relic or medal is now immersed in it, all those who will drink this water or who are blessed with it may have health in body and protection in soul; through Christ our Lord.

All: Amen.

Then the medal or relic is removed from the water. Then the following is said.

Let us pray. God, who through Blessed Vincent have added to your Church a new community to serve the poor and to train the clergy; grant, we pray, that we may be imbued with the same fervour, so as to love what he loved and to carry out what he taught; through Christ our Lord. Amen.

Recommended Reading

Pat Collins C.M. Writings on Healing

"Freedom from Addiction" in *Freedom from Evil Spirits: Released from Fear, Addiction and the Devil* (Dublin: Columba Books, 2019), 77-124.

"Praying for Healing" *Maturing in the Spirit: Guidelines for Prayer Groups* (Dublin: Columba Books, 1991), 125-140

"The Healing Power of Intimacy" *Intimacy and the Hungers of the Heart* (Dublin: Columba Books, 1991), 144-165.

"Forgiveness and Healing" *Growing in Health and Grace* (Galway: Campus, 1992), 7-26

"Faith and Eucharistic Healing" *Finding Faith in Troubled Times* (Dublin: Columba Books, 1993), 150-183.

"Freedom From Addiction" *Unveiling The Heart: How To Overcome Evil in the Christian Life* (Dublin: Veritas, 1995), 67-76

"Faith and the Anointing of the Sick" *Expectant Faith* (Dublin: Columba Books, 1998), 141-150.

"Prayer for Healing" *Spirituality for the 21st Century* (Dublin: Columba Books, 1999), 150-169.

"The Prayer of Command" *Prayer in Practice: A Biblical Approach* (Dublin: Columba Books, 2000), 148-166.

"Is Prayer Good for Your Health?" *Spirituality* (Sept/Oct 2001), 294-298; "Why Prayer is Good for Your Health" *Reality,* (Jan 2002), 21-22; "Is Prayer Good for Your Health?" *Broken Image: Reflections on Religion and Culture"* (Dublin: Columba Books, 2002), 86-92.

Reducing Stress and Finding Peace (Dublin: Veritas, 2002)

Some More Writings on Healing

Morton Kelsey *Healing & Christianity* (London: SCM, 1973)

Agnes Sanford *The Healing Light* (The Drift, Evesham: Arthur James, 1974)

Francis Mc Nutt *Healing* (Notre Dame, Ave Maria Press, 1974)

The Power to Heal (Notre Dame: Ave Maria Press, 1977)

Deliverance From Evil Spirits (London: Hodder & Stoughton, 1996)

The Nearly Perfect Crime: How the Church Almost Killed the Ministry of Healing (Grand Rapids: Chosen, 2005).

John Wimber *Power Healing* (London: Hodder & Stoughton, 1986)

Kenneth Mc Call *Healing the Family Tree* (London: Sheldon Press, 1994)

Jim Mc Manus *The Healing Power of the Sacraments* (Notre Dame: Ave Maria Press 1984)

Cardinal Ratzinger, "Instruction on Prayers for Healing" Congregation for the Doctrine of the faith (Sept 14th 2000).

Smith Wigglesworth, *Greater Works* (New Kensington, PA: Whitaker House,1999)

Damian Stayne, *Renew Your Wonders: Spiritual Gifts for Today* (Luton: New Life, 2017)

Sr Briege McKenna O.S.C., *Miracles Do Happen: God Can Do the Impossible* (Dublin: Veritas, 1987)

John Gunstone, *Healed, Restored, Forgiven: Liturgies, Prayers and Readings for the Ministry of Healing* (Norwich: Canterbury Press, 2004).

Heather Parsons, *Father Peter Rookey: Man of Miracles* (Dublin: Robert Andrew Press, 1994).

Andy O'Neill, *The Power of Charismatic Healing* (Irish American Book Co., 1998)

—— *The Miracle of Charismatic Healing* (Cork: Mercier Press, 1996).

—— *Charismatic Healing in Everyday Life* (Cork: Mercier Press, 1991).

Want to keep reading?

Columba Books has a whole range of books to inspire your faith and spirituality.

As the leading independent publisher of religious and theological books in Ireland, we publish across a broad range of areas including pastoral resources, spirituality, theology, the arts and history.

All our books are available through
www.columbabooks.com
and you can find us on Twitter, Facebook and Instagram to discover more of our fantastic range of books. You can sign up to our newletter through the website for the latest news about events, sales and to keep up to date with our new releases.

columbabooks

@ColumbaBooks

columba_books

columba
BOOKS

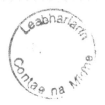